self-care for tough times

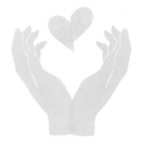

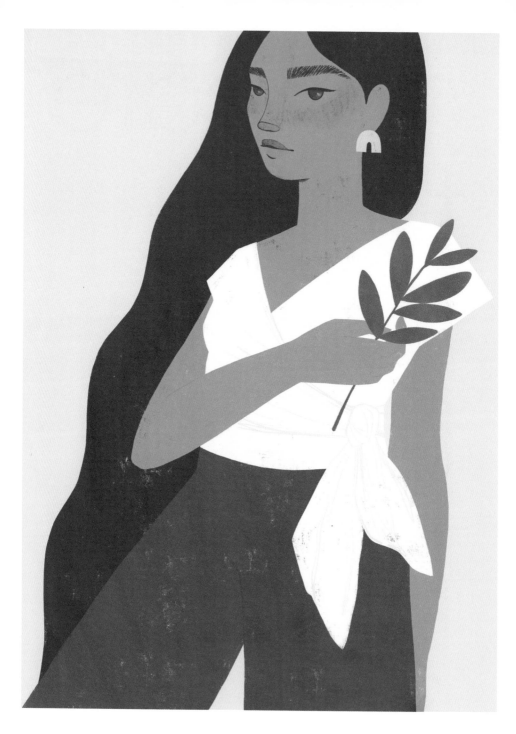

self-care for tough times

How to heal in times of anxiety, loss & change

Suzy Reading

For anyone in the midst of tough times, you're not alone.
We walk the healing path together.

An Hachette UK Company
www.hachette.co.uk

First published in Great Britain as an ebook in 2020 by Aster, an imprint of
Octopus Publishing Group Ltd
Carmelite House
50 Victoria Embankment
London EC4Y 0DZ
www.octopusbooks.co.uk

This edition published in 2021

Distributed in the US by
Hachette Book Group
1290 Avenue of the Americas
4th and 5th Floors
New York, NY 10104

Distributed in Canada by
Canadian Manda Group
664 Annette St.
Toronto, Ontario, Canada M6S 2C8

ISBN 978-1-78325-375-3

A CIP catalogue record for this book is available from the British Library.

Printed and bound in China

10 9 8 7 6 5 4 3 2 1

Consultant publisher: Kate Adams
Senior editor: Pauline Bache
Copyeditor: Katy Denny
Art director: Yasia Williams-Leedham
Illustrator: Madeline Kate Martinez
Production manager: Lisa Pinnell

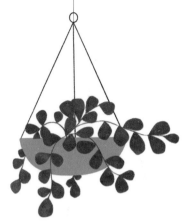

Contents

Introduction

Tough times. It's the receipt of news that sucks all the air from your lungs, making you wonder how you'll ever breathe again. It's the instant that changes your world completely, and the disconnect that arises from looking outside and seeing that life goes on as if nothing has happened. It's the staggering loss that words can never truly capture. It's the betrayal that cracks you open to your core. It's the first dawning that life is precarious, precious and ultimately finite, and that there really are no guarantees. It's in the daily grind, the pressure cooker of work life, family life, parenting and all the responsibilities we wear, consuming our life force. It can be something you wanted with all your heart, something you had to fight tenaciously for, but now it's yours, the reality of it is so much harder than you could ever have anticipated. It's also in the shades of grey where one life chapter closes and the next is yet to blossom. It's in the grief of a lost imagined future, even when you're actively choosing what lies ahead. It's in the milestones of life and all those firsts and lasts. The one unifying thought is wondering how you're going to get through this.

That's where our journey together begins.

Behind the public smiles that greet you in everyday life, beneath the filtered highlights you meet scrolling online, we are all vulnerable to tough times. No one is immune from challenging life experiences, big emotions, loss and times of real squeeze. We all go through tough times and if you feel floored in the midst of one or are still recovering from one, know that this doesn't mean you're weak, it means you're human.

What might surprise you is that when we start describing events that constitute 'tough times' there are a whole host of them that perhaps you hadn't really considered as being taxing; things that you desperately want, like moving, renovation projects or starting a family, things that you aspire to, like a promotion, launching your own business or buying your own home. Many of these things accumulate, they often coincide, and actually when we take a good look at what we've weathered, it's no wonder that we're left trembling in their wake. I hope that in reframing how we see these life events – by removing blame and self-flagellation – you will be able to have a greater sense of peace in your response to them and permission to do things differently during that stage, chapter or time of life. We're going to walk the healing path together and I'm going to empower you with a skill set that will see you through and help you restore yourself on the other side, before life inevitably calls on you to step up again.

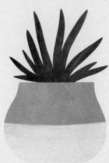

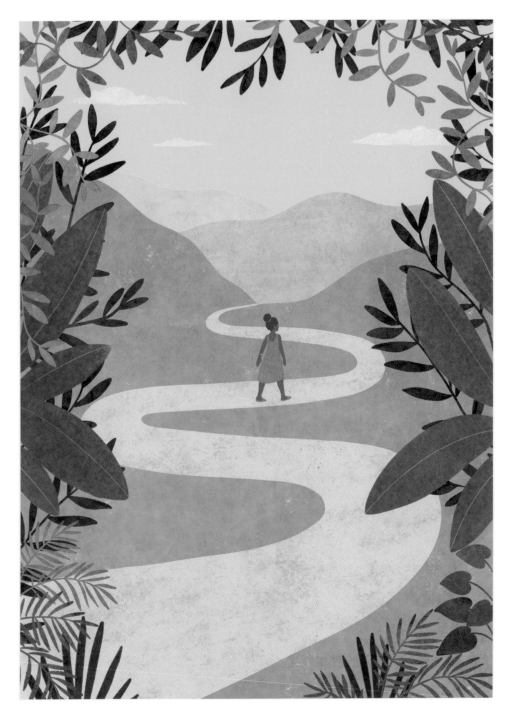

What are tough times? They come in many different guises: some desirable, some unwanted, and many are completely unavoidable. We all have a fallible mind and body, we all experience stress in our careers, family life and relationships and we all lose people we love. Broadly speaking, and this is informed by my work as a chartered psychologist and my own lived experience, there are three themes: there is stress and burnout, there is loss and grief and there is change and transition. Each of these experiences requires its own specific toolkit of *skills* to cope during, and to restore afterwards. Some occurrences in life will involve just one theme; others will involve all three. Often we struggle with an event without realizing we've incurred a loss. Just making this connection, acknowledging your loss, unlocks your own innate healing capacity. Recognition of how an experience can be affecting you and knowledge of ways to navigate stress, loss and change will put you in good stead for whatever life throws at you.

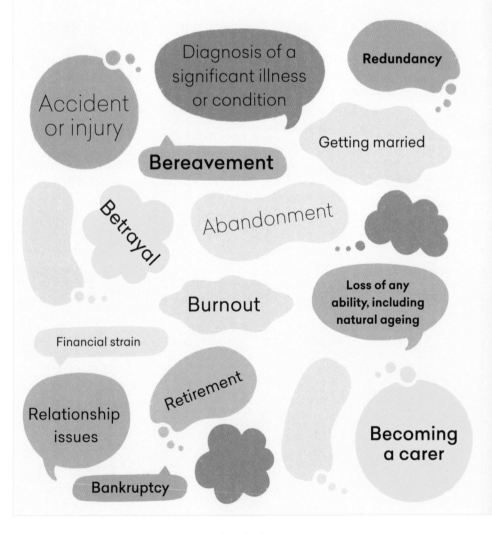

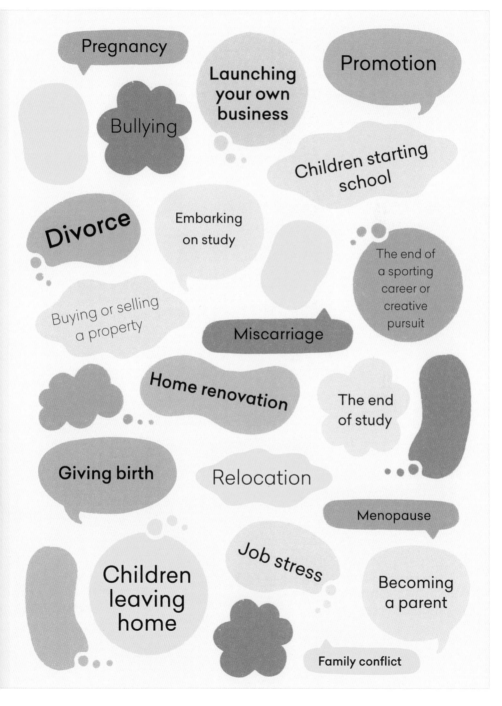

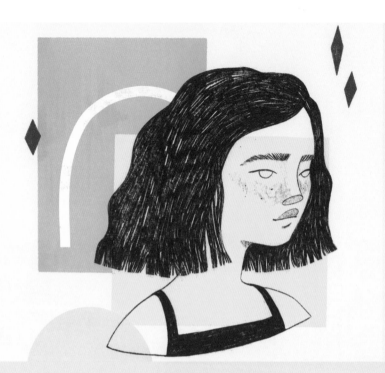

HOW THIS BOOK CAN HELP

If you're in the midst or the aftermath of any of these experiences, this book can help you cope, heal and restore. It can boost your resolve and resilience to help you prepare for an impending challenge. If you're a partner, parent, family member, friend or practitioner, it will give you greater insight so you can better understand and support others. We all stand to gain a great deal by talking openly about our experiences. Great healing, a deep sense of connection and true empowerment come from that honest dialogue. Let's get that ball rolling together.

Often it's not until crisis hits and we descend into energetic bankruptcy, that we truly appreciate our health and understand the genuine need for self-care. We begin to recognize it as the means to clawing back our health and what this facilitates in our life. We see it as the means to processing our swirling emotions and moving through challenging life events. We understand that if we don't nourish ourselves, we make ourselves vulnerable to burnout, anxiety and depression. That lived experience spurs us on to make different choices and self-care becomes a way of life, so that we can keep putting one foot in front of the other, because we know how hard it can be. If you're not there yet, it's ok. We'll acknowledge the barriers to self-care and I will show you how, little by little, you can imbue *today* with tenderness.

You might be feeling so bone tired that you don't know how you'll get out of bed, let alone tackle what's required of you. Maybe you're battling with emotions so enormous you fear they'll take over and the tears could never stop. Perhaps you feel so lost and confused that you don't know where to start or who you are any more. You might be wondering how everyone else manages to have it all together, when you feel like you're falling apart. The truth is, we are all struggling in our own ways. Don't compare how you feel inside with how others appear on the outside. What you see in real life is just the tip of the iceberg and just about everything you see on social media is someone's 'best bits'.

All these experiences can make you feel like you're losing your mind. I've lost count of the number of people I've heard voicing that terrifying concern. You are not alone. I've been there, I know how distant your health and vitality can feel and just how impossible self-care or any solution can seem.

Often when we find ourselves in tough times, the situation is compounded by self-care falling away. This is totally normal so please don't give yourself a hard time about it. Harsh criticism doesn't change your circumstances, it just adds to your burden. Compassion yields a far more effective outcome. But if that feels like a difficult habit to break, please don't worry, that's what this book is all about: developing a capacity for tenderness and forming new healthy habits that serve us. I will show you how to throw yourself a bone. It really is one of the greatest skills in life.

The fact is when we need self-care the most, that's when it's often the hardest to do. That's what happened to me. My whole career revolved around health-promoting strategies – I was (and still am) a chartered psychologist, yoga teacher and personal trainer. I had every nourishing tool at my fingertips, but this was my first real experience of being seriously tested by life. I became a mum at the same time as losing my dad and no degree or training really prepares you for a collision of life events like that. Self-care is relatively simple when life is smooth.

When we get squeezed by life it can be so hard to find ways to nurture ourselves, that's if we've cottoned on to the fact that we are not invincible and the machinery that we're comprised of requires tender, loving attention. For so many of us, self-care feels out of reach because we're too pressed for time, bereft of energy, out of ideas on things that feel do-able, and the most tenacious barrier of all is guilt. We feel guilty taking time for us because it diverts resources from other precious people or responsibilities.

What I learned the hard way was that denying my needs, relentlessly pushing on and ignoring my health, and steadfastly believing in my invincibility, lead me to one place only – energetic rock bottom. And in that place I was no good to anyone. To be the mum, wife, family member, friend and practitioner that I aspired to be, I had to take nourishing action. This is the realization that helps us make peace with guilt, to allow it to be there and take care of ourselves in the face of it. And that learning dropped in even deeper when life tested me again – unbelievably with the same variables – international relocation, having a child and bereavement, rolled into one sucker punch. Second time round was a vastly different experience. It was still deeply challenging and painful at times, but my new relationship with self-care, a profound awareness of its importance and an extensive toolkit sustained me and had me back to firing on all cylinders much faster.

Many of us find ourselves overwhelmed by tough times because we haven't been empowered with the tools to navigate them. There is great solace in embracing the knowledge that it's not your fault. Please let those words linger. Raised in a culture of being told to 'get up, dust yourself off, you're ok, don't cry' and the notion of the 'stiff upper lip' meant that as children many of us were traditionally discouraged from expressing our emotions, so it's no wonder that we struggle with stress, loss and change as adults. And now the pendulum has swung too far the other way and we see 'helicopter parents' trying to save their kids from experiencing the teensiest bit of discomfort or tricky emotion. If we tie our kid's shoelaces all the time, we hamper their development of that skill; similarly, if we rush in to 'fix' situations or quell emotions, we can get in the way of empowering problem-solving skills, emotional agility and confidence. The fact is, many of these skills have not been modelled for us and we are now learning together.

Modern culture also prizes intellect while negating the wisdom of the body. In fact we still spend a great deal of energy learning how to override what the body naturally wants us to do. Remember how hard it was to sit still in school? I bet you still feel that now at your desk if you get really quiet and listen. It took great effort to stamp out those impulses and tune out the messages from our bodies. We need to reclaim the right to feel, the ability to feel what we feel, to give voice and move through our emotions with tenderness and self-compassion.

Your body has an innate capacity to restore itself to health. You are biologically designed to heal. I'm here to help you reconnect with this natural ability, to help you get out of your own way so you can facilitate the healing process, by adopting life-giving habits rather than coping mechanisms or crutches that only feel good in the short term. Essentially this is about unlocking your self-soothing capacity and learning how to manage your energy. Together we will look at the skills that help us weather stress, loss and change. We will revive a weary body. We will refresh a tired mind. We will heal your broken heart. We will mobilize your inner healing resources and get you back to vitality and clarity.

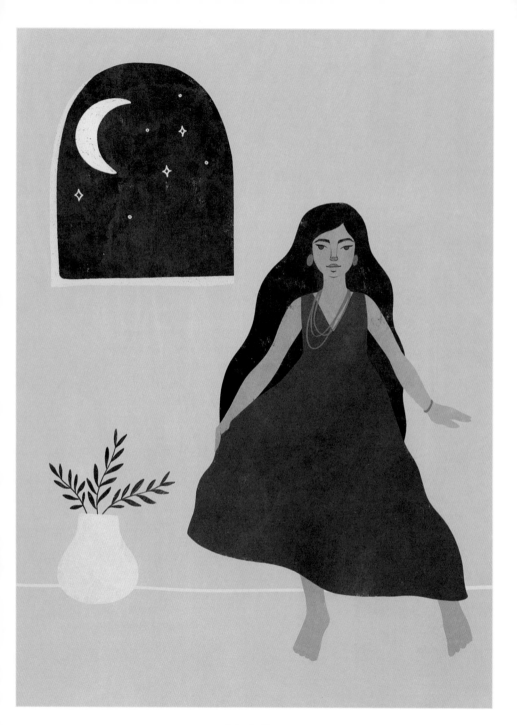

What is self-care all about?

Self-care has become a buzzword of late. There are good reasons for this rise in awareness, although there is genuinely nothing new about the concept. The term was used originally in the context of people working in high-stress occupations – therapists, medical practitioners and those at the forefront of the emergency services. Contrary to what you might read in the papers, that it's just a fad or that it's wellbeing gone overboard, the practice is here to stay. As a society we are beginning to engage in a more open dialogue about mental health and we are increasingly aware of the need for strategies to help us cope better during tough times. There is a growing concern about how we can nourish our mental and emotional health because the statistics are alarming, especially in our young people. With figures like 'a quarter of 14-year-old girls in the UK have self-harmed'[1], and studies showing that emotional disorders in children are on the increase, where one in eight (12.8 per cent) 5- to 19-year-olds had at least one mental disorder when assessed in 2017[2], we simply can't

afford to be dismissive of self-care or complacent about empowering our kids with these life-giving skills.

The tragic rate of suicide in men (17.2 deaths per 100,000 in 2018[3]), the fact that suicide is the leading cause of death in new mothers[4] and the coinciding increase of suicide over the period of life where women are likely to go through menopause[5] is further evidence that we need to take urgent action.

While there might be some confusion about what self-care is and some valid opposition to the term being hijacked by brands trying to tout their beauty products, there really is nothing fluffy or indulgent about self-care. It is rising to prominence now because of the growing body of research into mindfulness, resilience, compassion and other health-promoting skills. In the late Nineties there was a paradigm shift in psychology where the focus changed from examining mental illness to looking at the foundations of wellbeing. We've had two decades of rigorous scientific study into what makes life worth living and this forms the backbone to the strategies we'll explore together in this book.

WHAT REALLY IS SELF-CARE?

The simplest definition I can offer is *self-care is health care*. It is nourishing all layers of your being – your mental health, your physical health and your emotional health, all of which are inextricably linked. To get crystal clear on what is truly nourishing we need to take into consideration the immediate and long-term consequences – so self-care is something that nurtures you right now, *and* promotes your health in the future, nourishing your 'future self'. This can be a useful distinction to make and will help you see the difference between a crutch and a genuine self-care solution. Another way to understand self-care is to think of it as energy management. We need energy to get through our day and the healthier our energetic bank balance, the better prepared we are when life gets tough. Regular deposits into our energy bank via self-care boost our ability to cope in the moment and to bounce back faster.

WHAT DOES SELF-CARE LOOK LIKE?

In reality self-care takes many different shapes because different things appeal to different people. Your own preferences change over time too, so you'll need different things in different moments and that's why we all need an extensive, personalized toolkit. Self-care can be singing in a choir, fishing, painting, journalling, dancing or socializing, but equally it can be feeling your breath, a word of gratitude as you sit to eat your evening meal, tasting the flavours, noticing the sensation of sunlight on your skin as you drive to work or imbibing the scent as you fold the freshly laundered washing. Most people associate self-care with some kind of practice or ritual and this is a natural assumption, but I want to broaden that thinking.

Self-care is not only an act, it is also a set of skills. The beauty is that when you develop these skills you can apply them to everyday actions, to life as it unfolds. Self-care is then no longer something added to your already jampacked 'to do' list – it is a lens through which you experience life, transforming the way you respond to it.

These skills help us reframe and interpret events more constructively, reducing our stress levels, keeping us calm and anchored, and they open us up to experiencing more moments of joy and peace. As these skills become embedded in our day as habits, self-care becomes a way of life, not an extra thing to be done. We can remove the barrier of 'not enough time'! While I will be sharing many nourishing activities in this book, at the heart of them all is the development of these key skills. These are skills you are already in possession of, but just naming them makes them more salient. They're just like muscles and they will strengthen and grow as we put them to good use.

The benefits of self-care

- Self-care helps us cope in the moment during tough times.

- Self-care helps us recover and heal after challenging experiences or chapters of life.

- Self-care boosts our resilience, giving us some protection from future stress and helps us bounce back quicker.

- Self-care gives us access to an incarnation of ourselves we can take pride in, benefitting every person with whom we come into contact.

- Self-care boosts the health of our relationships, family harmony and helps us raise emotionally aware, fully empowered kids.

MAKING SELF-CARE POSSIBLE DURING TOUGH TIMES

In the midst of stress, loss and change we need a whole new nourishing toolkit. The things that we habitually turn to when life is smooth often become out of reach or just don't meet our needs in this time of challenge. Getting to our favourite yoga class feels too much, going out for that run feels like wading through treacle, even seeing friends you love can feel exhausting. In this brain fog it is also really hard to put your finger on something do-able, so we often turn to coffee to get us going, food and alcohol to numb us and screens to distract us. These might help us manage in the short term but they won't truly sustain us or do us any favours in the long term. The toll these crutches have on our sleep alone creates an even bigger deficit to address. This book will give you many life-giving options to choose from. Things that take no time. Things that require no energy. Things that don't cost a penny. Together, we will find a way.

Before we launch ahead, let's ponder a while. Please do this with as much tenderness as possible. Judgement and self-criticism just get in the way. What's done is done, and we now have a choice as to how we proceed.

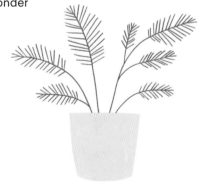

1. What are the things that you are turning to right now for comfort and support? Are they genuinely tending to your needs in the moment and are they nurturing your future self? At what cost do you keep using these coping mechanisms?

2. Are there some soothing pursuits that you've forgotten about? Is there something you would like to reclaim? Maybe you'd like to pick up your guitar again or is there a place you'd like to go and sit to feel connected with someone? Perhaps you'd like to return to something but it needs to take a different shape now with your current life variables. How can you dip into it in a way that honours where you are at right now? If you can't think of a way, sit down with a friend and see if together you can find one, or something new that helps you meet that need.

3. Thinking of self-care as energy management, give yourself permission to guard your precious energy bank. Are there energy zappers that you can eliminate, avoid or minimize? Identify those people, places or tasks that deplete you and think of steps you can take to protect yourself. If these energy zappers are unavoidable, use this book to top up your energy bank in compensation.

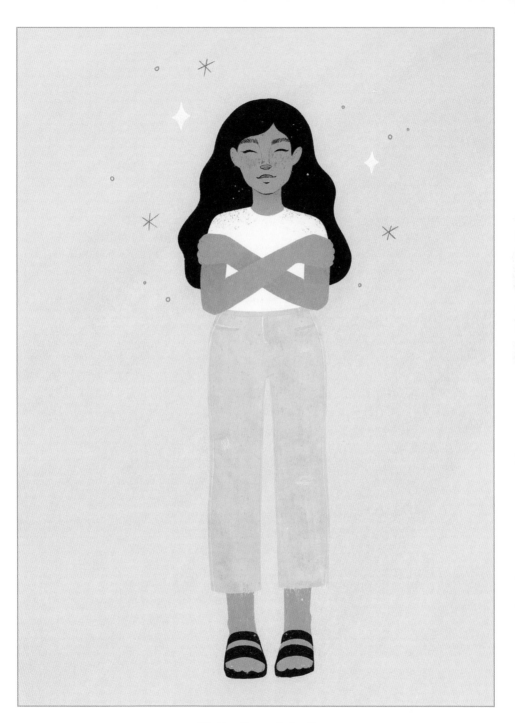

What is self-care all about?

WHY SELF-CARE CAN BE SO HARD

It's more than just the time, energy and expense conundrum. Self-care is health care, and we all know what we need to do to be healthy, right? But this stuff is not easy. The healthy choice is not always the most alluring. Sometimes the real act of self-care is uncomfortable! Self-care certainly isn't always pampering, sometimes it is the last thing you feel like doing, but it is the thing that will help you heal and your future self will thank you for it. I think it's really important to point this out. If you're struggling with it, cut yourself some slack. We all struggle with this. Don't let this be another stick you beat yourself with and there is no failing at it. There is just the opportunity to learn and make different choices.

If the healthy choice is hard at the best of times, let's recognize how tough it can be in times of crisis. It is hard to delay gratification when our willpower reserves are at rock bottom, when we're in the throes of decision-making fatigue or just too exhausted or grief-stricken to be able to think straight. When we're at the ransom of stress hormones, the heaviness of grief, the confusion of change, a state of sleep deprivation, in physical or emotional pain, it can be incredibly hard to think with clarity and act with purpose. Where possible, observing the 'energy bank basics' will help you make more constructive choices – getting adequate sleep, feeding your mind and body, making sure you're well watered, spending time in nature and in connection with other people, and moving for mental health. I completely understand that our access to these very things is impinged on during tough times, but this book will show you how to make it possible. Please go gently on yourself and know that we all tend to rely on crutches to get us through. I certainly did and I still find those old habits creep in, until I get a warning sign from my body and mind to take different action.

HOW TO OVERCOME GUILT

You might find that guilt keeps popping up and stopping you in your tracks, or even deeper than that, a feeling that you don't deserve to feel better. Let's be clear: every human being deserves to feel nourished. Every human being is worthy of love and care. Regardless of what you've been told or how you've been made to feel, and if this is speaking to you, my heart goes out to you – *you deserve to feel loved and cared for.*

To make peace with these feelings, take a moment to connect with your personal 'why' of self-care. This is the stuff that will truly free you and motivate you to take alternative action, because if you want to feel differently, you've got to do things differently. It's not enough just to think about it.

1. Think about one role in life that feels really important to you. It could be partner, parent, carer, business owner or practitioner. Reflect on the kind of qualities you aspire to possess in this role. How do you want to be experienced? What kind of behaviour and values do you want to model? What kind of legacy would you like to leave?

2. Now jot down the kind of scaffolding you need in life to be able to be this version of you, being as specific as you can, from morning through till evening. What are the non-negotiables in everyday life necessary for you to be able to function in this way?

3. Based on your reflections to the prompts above, write down what self-care facilitates in your life, for you and your loved ones. Write down why it's not only ok but necessary to do it. Return to this list whenever guilt gets in the way.

Notice how the benefits of self-care ripple out far beyond you as an individual and remember this the next time guilt taps you on the shoulder. It needn't be narcissistic in nature at all, it's simply acknowledging that your needs should get a look in too. Your health is important too. It's not me 'first', it's me 'as well' and this is the stuff that allows us to weather the tough times, to get back on our feet and to show up in this world as our heart's desire.

HOW CAN WE GET REAL, PRACTICAL SELF-CARE ON THE RADAR?

The simplest and quickest way to connect with something nourishing when we need it the most is to refer to a diagram, and that's why I created The Vitality Wheel. The Vitality Wheel is like a mind map and I hope it broadens what you think of as self-care. It is far more than bubble baths, pedicures and weekend breaks. The Vitality Wheel will show you the eight different ways that you can top up your energy bank. Most of this will not be new to you, but maybe you haven't associated some of the spokes of the wheel with self-care. It also serves to remind you, because when we're feeling overwhelmed, this is the knowledge that's really hard to call to mind. Rather than running through a long list of self-care ideas, if you annotate the wheel with the same inspiration, you will locate it far more quickly – swiftly putting your finger on something resonant and accessible right now.

Keep your wheel on the fridge, in your diary, next to your bed and it will help you take more nourishing action, more often, and this is how we cope and how we heal. Each section of this book will give you plenty of fresh inspiration to add to your wheel. Add the mantras that speak to you, the yoga poses that hit the spot, the breathing exercises, coping tools or ways to channel the therapeutic power of nature. Some things will resonate now, some might not and that's fine. This is not a 'one size fits all' approach. But what I will say is that things change quickly and our toolkit serves us best when we

THE VITALITY WHEEL PATHWAYS

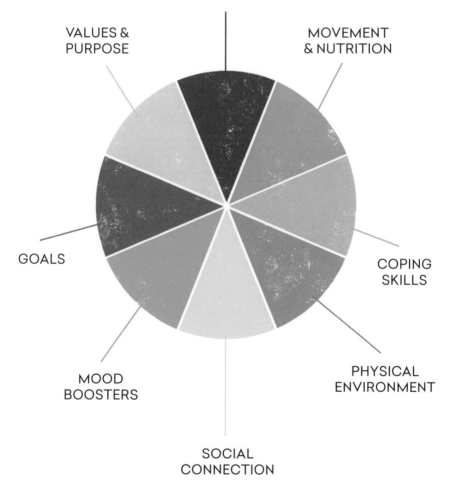

SLEEP, REST, RELAXATION & BREATHING

MOVEMENT & NUTRITION

VALUES & PURPOSE

GOALS

COPING SKILLS

MOOD BOOSTERS

PHYSICAL ENVIRONMENT

SOCIAL CONNECTION

keep it evolving. Keep checking in with this book and let your wheel evolve too. Turn to your wheel when you need a boost, when you need to wind down or when you have a precious spare minute. Use your diary to set aside some time for your replenishment by making an appointment with you and use the wheel to identify the best choice in the moment.

MY HEARTFELT WISH FOR THIS BOOK

Tough times hurt, there is no getting around it, but I am hoping this book can help you through it. I'll draw on my own lived experience of navigating stress, loss and change – and share with you the normal, fallible human side of things, and I'll call on my professional experience as a chartered psychologist, qualified yoga teacher and personal trainer, so you know that research backs up this toolkit. My intention is to impart soothing tonics using the body, touch, breath, movement and the mind, all of which tap into broader skills that guide you through life:

» **to come home to your body**

» **to be your own safe place**

» **to reclaim the ability to relax and replenish**

» to understand your emotions, develop the ability to identify them, give voice to them and move through them, even the ones you are scared will break you

» to awaken your deep self-soothing capacity

» to remind you that you have your own back, you can speak your truth and honour your boundaries

» to strengthen you so you have the patience to tolerate ambiguity and times of confusion

» to develop self-insight, knowledge of your greatest strengths, your values and your purpose. These will give you clarity, guide you and motivate you as you carve your path forward and embark on a new path imbued with tenderness, kindness and compassion

HOW TO JOURNEY THROUGH THIS BOOK

There are three main sections of this book: the first deals with stress and burnout, the second addresses loss and grief and the third examines change and transition. You can read the book cover to cover or you can head straight to the section that calls to you most, dipping in just where you feel drawn. If you can only manage a page a time, that's fine. If you just want to look at the pictures, that's a great starting point too. In the midst of life's challenges take the path of least resistance and don't expect too much of yourself. Reading just one mantra or paragraph might just help create a shift. We will explore what each theme looks like, the effect it can have on us and the specific toolkit we can draw upon to help us through it. We will start with super simple practices and build to more elaborate or challenging ideas, each of which plants a seed of *skill acquisition:*

STRESS & BURNOUT » this is about reclaiming connection with your body, the ability to relax, the skill of physically letting go, and understanding how to restore, re-energize and replenish. If you're exhausted, if you want to release physical burden or find calm, this is the place to start.

LOSS & GRIEF » this is about feeling your feelings, emotional expression and release, giving voice and self-soothing. Start here if you want to let go of your emotional burden, if your mood is low or you're in emotional pain.

CHANGE & TRANSITION » this is about making peace with uncertainty and developing tolerance for the discomfort of change, the skill of equanimity which builds on the skills we explore in the first two sections. This section is also about self-insight and the inner work of change. Think of this as your 'what to do next' section, carving a plan of action and setting goals. Start here when you feel sufficient energy to take action, if you're confused and want clarity or if you want to feel greater peace.

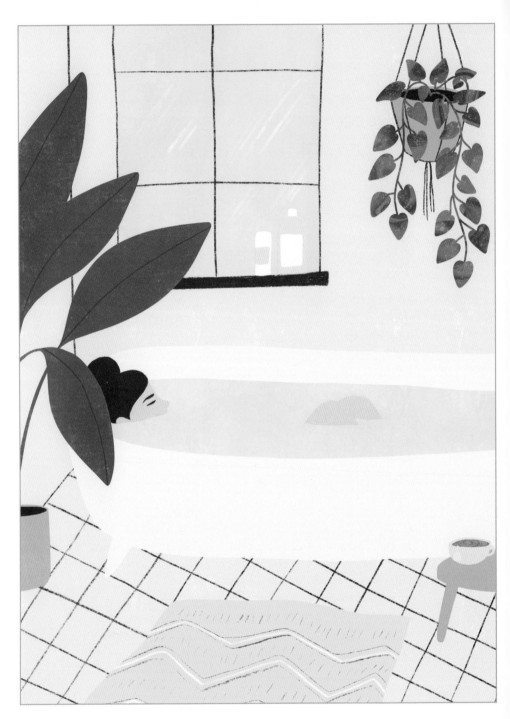

What is self-care all about?

THE SCOPE OF SELF-CARE & THIS BOOK

I am an advocate for self-care, but this is not about doing it all on your own. We all need support, a sense of belonging, loving connection. We need other people to help us cope and heal, to be seen and heard, understood and validated, to be held. While I want to empower you with tonics and skills, I also want to encourage you to reach out. I needed to draw on the strength of others, the love and support of those dear to me and professional support. I still rely on that net of love and care around me now in smoother times. This book is not a substitute for counselling, the healing that comes from being in a therapeutic *relationship*, but is intended to empower you with tools in addition to the support of people around you.

While it's not about doing it all by yourself, self-care is about *self-responsibility*. It is stepping up, taking ownership of your life, and choosing life-giving action over sticking your head in the sand or opting for something that just numbs or distracts you. It is acknowledging that you are responsible for your health, your actions and how you respond to life. There's no point wishing tough times away, they're happening whether you like it or not. Terrible things happen to the most loving, people. There is no justice. You don't deserve this. But at the end of the day, it is happening and there's no point denying it or waiting for someone else to come and rescue you. You have to deal with the variables you're facing and all you can do is choose how you respond. While that involves allowing ourselves the time and space for a normal, human reaction, which may be justifiable rage and total overwhelm, there will come a moment when things click and you'll feel ready to take action, to hope that things can get better or you'll make damn certain that the time left is to be prized and used to the full. I hope that this book can be the friend in your back pocket, willing you on and empowering you with things that you can do to help you through this tough time and to promote healing on the other side.

You might flip through the pages of this book and wonder how on earth a single yoga pose or something as simple as holding your own hand could possibly help you through this heartache. I think that's a very fair question, but understand the potency of these practices lies in the intention with which you imbue the action – it's about planting a seed that will deepen your innate healing potential. Each simple practice sets out to develop an ability that you already possess, but by drawing awareness to its value and by practising it, we further develop those skills, just as we build a muscle. These practices also have a cumulative effect so by dotting them through our day, their healing power grows. Even if in isolation these practices don't seem ground-breaking, understand that they at least provide you with an alternative to less health-promoting choices that we otherwise habitually turn to – like comfort eating or zoning out with screens. I also hope that these soothing rituals will provide you with some welcome distraction from worry, overthinking and negativity. This book will empower you with things that you can actually do to make a difference. Maybe we can't change the hand you've been dealt but this book can help you break free from feeling like a passive recipient of life and to respond with more constructive, life-giving action.

It's about planting a seed that will deepen your innate healing potential.

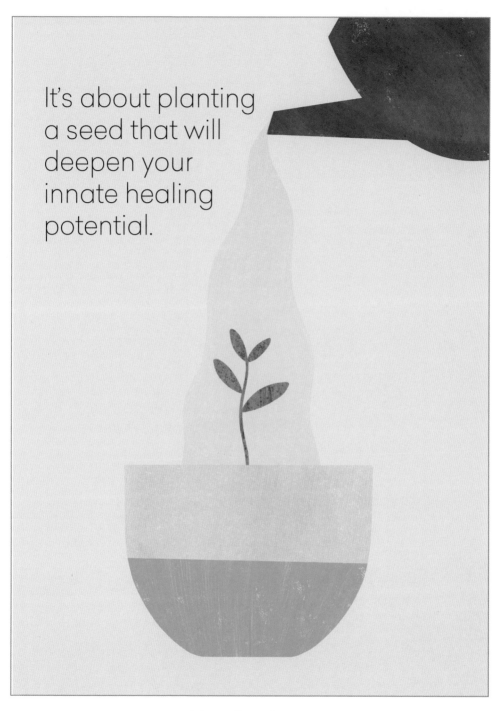

A NOTE ON TRAUMA:
YOU ARE STUCK, NOT BROKEN

A little caveat here, my intention for this book is to support you through tough times. It is beyond the scope of this book to resolve trauma. To heal from trauma we need to be in a relationship with another person, someone who can provide a feeling of safety and a container to hold you as you bear the reality of your experience. Restoring relationships and connection is central to restoring wellbeing[6]. You need to feel cared about, to have someone to truly count on, reminding you of your shared humanity. The effects of trauma are found in the emotional brain and nervous system and we need to be guided by a practitioner who is trauma aware, to facilitate the necessary physiological rewiring. It's not enough to try to change the way we think because the effects of trauma lie beneath conscious control.

While that partnered therapy is not possible through the pages of this book, what I do want you to know if you are feeling traumatized, is that you are not broken. You are just stuck. I felt broken too, but it's not irrevocable. Healing is possible. Peter Levine, trauma expert, sums it up beautifully: 'Trauma is a fact of life. It does not however need to be a life sentence'[7]. You can come home to your body. You can feel safe in your body again. You can retrain your nervous system to dial down the threat response and find peace in the present moment again. You can learn to calm and relax and develop a caring relationship with yourself. You can reconnect with your personal power, energy and courage. You can rekindle a feeling of agency and take charge of your life. Please seek out someone trained and experienced in trauma to partner you on that healing journey and I hope the practices in this book can augment that process.

Trauma 101

No one is immune from traumatic experiences and sadly it is happening all around us in loss, conflict and abuse, affecting not only those who are directly exposed to it but those around them at home, work, in the community, and impacting on subsequent generations as well. It is not only caused by significant events; we can feel traumatized by a series of events, big or small, and these are totally subjective. Sources include childhood experiences, medical procedures, giving birth, being involved in or witnessing accidents or natural disasters, violence, bullying and crime. An understanding of how trauma affects the brain and nervous system is helpful for everyone, allowing us to better understand ourselves, other people and to be compassionate in response. I particularly love Levine's call to reframe 'Post Traumatic Stress Disorder' to 'Post Traumatic Stress Injury' – PTSD is not anyone's fault, it's a normal (although disrupted) response to an extreme experience and we incur an injury as a result, a wound that can be healed.

These are some of the signs and symptoms of trauma:

» rage, irritability, mood swings, defensiveness

» shock, denial and disbelief

» numbing and emotional distance, feeling dead inside

» difficulty empathizing and engaging in close relationships, a fundamental distrust of yourself and others

» guilt, a sense of shame about something you've done or failure to act, self-blame

» anxiety and fear

» an altered sense of perception of the present moment, flashbacks, reliving memories, nightmares. Memories of past trauma can have the same effect on the brain as if the traumatic event is happening right now

» after trauma, the world is experienced with a different nervous system, feeling stuck in survival mode. Unresolved trauma causes people to respond excessively to the current situation. The internal alarm system keeps sending signals long after the danger is over, resulting in hypervigilance or numbing, disconnection and fragmentation. The rational brain can help us understand why we feel these things but it can't stop these sensations from occurring

» a feeling of being robbed of hope or a better future

How does trauma occur?

When we feel threatened there are five stages of response. These are valid survival mechanisms and they are all biologically wired responses, not conscious choices. Each stage reverts to a more primitive level of functioning and the more primitive the level of functioning, the more the evolved brain functions are suppressed. Interestingly, the way we heal is through this same hierarchy in reverse.

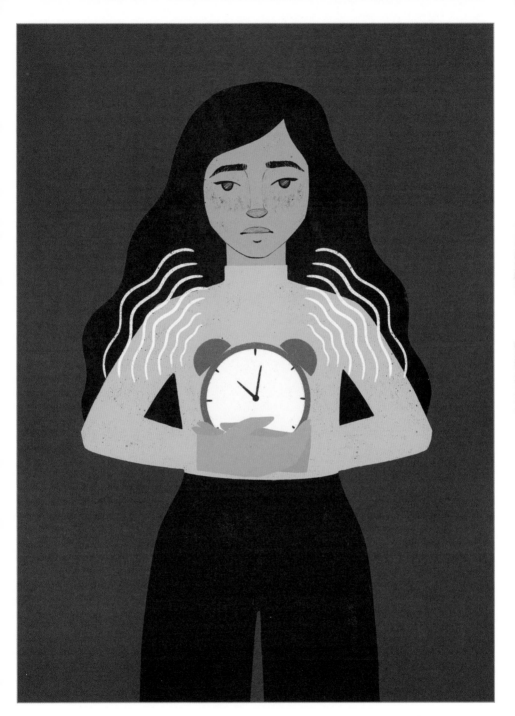

What is self-care all about?

After a threat this is the sequential order of response[8]

» ARREST – we pause to scan the environment to seek out danger. We are on the lookout. At this stage we draw on the 'social engagement system' by calling out for help or reassurance. This state is controlled by the ventral vagal complex, part of the parasympathetic nervous system, and in this state it is possible to remain calm, present and empathize with others.

If help is not at hand, then...

» FLIGHT – we try to escape the danger. The sympathetic nervous system now takes over and this state is characterized by restlessness, anxiety or fear. The more a person becomes engaged in flight, the more the prefrontal cortex goes offline and the older limbic brain kicks in, making us less capable of being calm or empathetic.

If escape is not possible, then...

» FIGHT – we get ready to defend ourselves. This state is also governed by the sympathetic nervous system and is characterized by irritability, anger or rage and we experience the same loss of cortical function as in flight.

If fighting won't protect us, then...

» FREEZE – it's possible we won't be seen if we're still and predators are less likely to eat something motionless, expending as little energy as possible in case there is another opportunity for fight or flight. This state is also governed by the vagal complex but a much more primitive part called the dorsal vagal complex.

If the freeze response isn't enough to protect us, then...

» FLOP – we collapse, triggering physiological numbing so pain and terror are dulled like a natural analgesic and dissociation helps us to bear the unbearable. Still mediated by the dorsal vagal complex, this is the last port of call for self-preservation.

Trauma arises when we're intensely frightened and either physically restrained or feel we're trapped. We either freeze in fear or collapse in helplessness. It is this complete immobility coupled with intense fear that creates trauma. When there's an overwhelming threat but no escape, the biological response is to shut down. If the individual survives, it's meant to be a temporary state but for humans we can get stuck in this response and show a tendency to freeze or an exaggerated vigilance to threat, where a non-traumatized person might only feel danger or excitement. If we've escaped danger by using flight or fight, we've been able to take action to free ourselves, thereby fully acting out the survival energy triggered by the threat. When we emerge from an experience of threat, via freeze or flop, we'll still have had the same impulses to run or fight, but these have been thwarted and we need to re-enact these movements or self-protective actions to discharge the survival energy and reset the nervous system. Acting out micro-movements, shaking or trembling is a way of discharging this survival energy. This is something animals instinctively do, but in humans, our logical, more evolved brain interferes with this primitive process. Levine postulates that to heal from trauma we need to gradually touch in with the immobilization response and to discharge the energy mobilized for life-preserving action.

If our survival actions are thwarted, they remain embedded in the body. If our guts and muscles are set to respond to danger, then our mind tells us there is something to fear and we'll keep searching for it, trapping us in the stress response. We're stuck on high alert, tense, on edge, fired up because our bodies are signalling danger to our brains. And you can imagine how utterly exhausting this is. If we stay on high alert long enough, lethargy, chronic fatigue, depression and a host of other conditions like IBS, migraines and fibromyalgia can result. It is quite possible that trauma lies at the heart of many modern illnesses.

What's important to note here is that all of these five responses are valid survival mechanisms. They are sequential and biologically driven. If the first strategy doesn't bring us to safety, our nervous system moves us to the next and so on. We do not consciously choose how we respond. This is crucially important in releasing people from guilt, shame or judgement for not fighting back in the moment. It is not weakness. It is not cowardice. And once traumatized, if someone remains hypervigilant or undervigilant, again this is not under voluntary control, it is a reflexive state. Do not blame the one who is over-sensitive to a perceived threat, or the one who freezes and fails to fight off a real threat. It is wired in our physiology, not intentional behaviour. Blame or shame are completely inappropriate and yelling at someone in this state will only further traumatize them. Stephen Porges offers us this powerful definition of trauma: 'it is chronic disruption of connectedness'[9]. Bessel van der Kolk sums it up for us: to resolve trauma one must 'know what you know and feel what you feel'[10], telling our truth even when that truth is painful, and the difficult task of learning to feel safe again. This is no small undertaking and it's a process that needs to be gently and expertly guided by an experienced therapist.

Yoga & its therapeutic properties

Leafing through the pages of this book you'll see lots of yoga poses. If you've never done yoga before, have no interest in yoga or feel it's not for you, please stick with me. If 'yoga' doesn't resonate, think of it as exercise or stretching, bringing the body into different shapes to create some kind of strengthening or releasing effect. All these exercises bring you into a closer relationship with your body, helping you get reacquainted, because you cannot muscle your way through tough times by staying in your head. You have to come home to your body to cope and heal.

When you look at the skill set of learning how to relax and let go, to feel what you feel and to be your own safe place – these are all held in the body, a visceral knowing. It doesn't help to intellectualize these things. They are a felt sense, anchored in our nervous system, the cells and fibres of our muscles, our posture, the freedom of the body to move and support itself. To weather tough times we need to draw on the mind, the breath, the body, movement and touch. Yoga is the perfect vehicle for this learning.

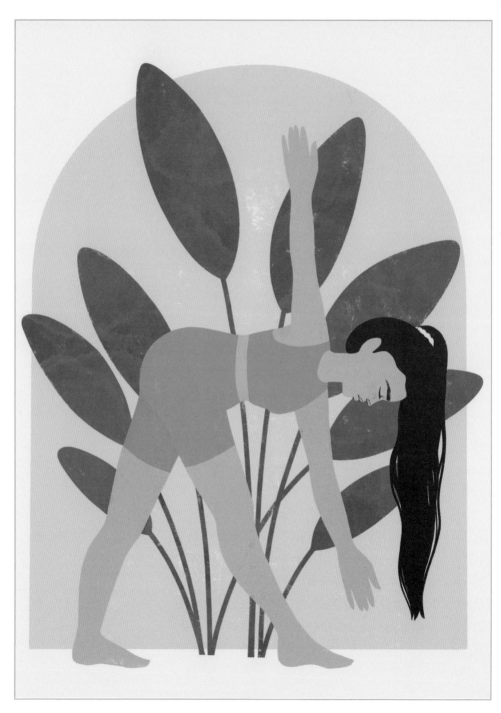

Yoga & its therapeutic properties

I'm not talking about yoga in the regular sense of going to a group class and spending an hour on the mat. I'm referring to simple practices that you can do on the sofa, in bed, on the floor, standing in the kitchen or sitting at your desk. Often it will be one pose at a time, or cobbling together a few into a sequence, if that feels good to you. This book will gently guide you. Whatever your ability, age, fitness level or state of flexibility, there will be accessible yoga in this book. Broadly speaking, the gentlest yoga will be found in the stress and loss sections and the more demanding will be found in the section on change. The practices in each section start out with minimal effort, energy or skill required and will get progressively more challenging. You can progress as you best see fit, honouring how you feel on the day. Every day will be different.

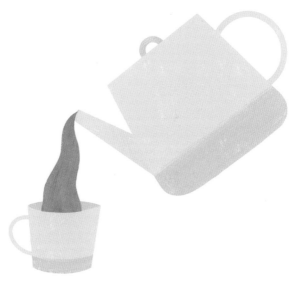

HOW DOES YOGA HELP?

Let me share with you my lived experience. This was my visceral response to witnessing my father's battle with motor neurone disease: I felt a vice-like tightening in my throat, a huge lump that wouldn't go away. I imagine it was all those things I couldn't say. I wanted his suffering, our suffering, to be over, but couldn't bring those words to the surface for the awful reality of what they meant. My emotional pain hung about my ribcage with such a heaviness that it shortened my every breath. When I sat still and tried to breathe deeper, it just made me feel more agitated because there was nowhere for it to go. It felt stuck and I felt stuck. Moving my body in time with my breath was the tonic. That was when the heaviness lifted and the constriction eased. I could feel the space between my ribs again, some sense of freedom in my breath. And the mantra is: *when you breathe better you feel better*.

Gentle yoga movement helped me reclaim the ability to breathe more fully, and this transformed how it felt to be in my body and how I moved through life.

Maybe you've been to a yoga class and felt a ripple of emotion wash through your body. I remember being overwhelmed by tears with no real catalyst in one of my early experiences of yoga. At the time I was foxed by it, but with gentle reassurance from my teacher I came to see this as a real gift. I want you to know that this is very normal and to be welcomed, but perhaps we need to take baby steps for it to feel safe, and that's ok. This book is based on baby steps that we take together. Yoga helps us release more than physical tension; there is an opportunity for emotional release that requires no further examination or digging, it can just be a wordless release, a profound letting go, when you're ready. Learning how to soften into a yoga pose, to make peace and sit with a difficult sensation, helped me navigate my loss. Fluid yoga, moving with the breath, helped me move through my grief and still helps me ride the waves nearly a decade later.

To be completely honest with you, in those very early days of motherhood, when I was energetically at my lowest, I used to roll out my yoga mat and sleep on it. Sleep, rest and stillness were what my body and mind were crying out for, so that's what I did. (In the weeks prior to that, I found myself watching daytime soaps and if you're not depressed before you watch them, you will be afterwards! I was lucky that my counsellor asked me the question 'What did you used to do to nourish yourself?' Yoga was always my tonic but now it had to take a very different shape. The lesson there was choose my downtime mindfully. Not all leisure activities are nourishing!)

With the baby monitor by my side, I'd set myself up with bolsters, cushions and blankets and settle into a restorative yoga pose. I knew my baby was safe and I could give myself permission to let go and rest. There was no pressure to drop off to sleep, as we feel when we hop

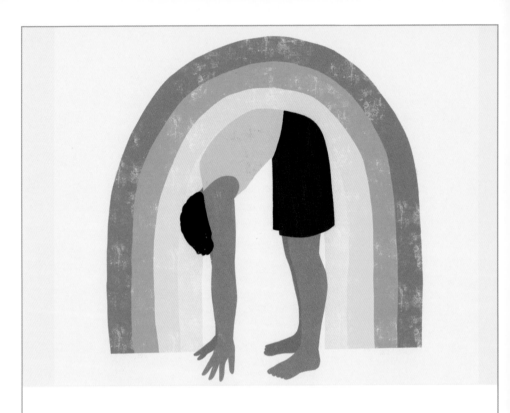

into bed for a nap. If I dozed off, it was a bonus. It didn't really matter if my cherub woke up after a short stint because even just a few minutes of lying down, held by the floor and support of the props beneath me, I knew I'd had some benefit. I lay down and slept on my yoga mat for months until there was a resurgence of energy and it felt time to move.

Initially, yoga was the way I replenished my energy bank, and moved through my emotions, then it literally got me back on my feet again. The next step of my healing journey was to build on that connection with my body and breath, to feel the grounding of my feet, the strength of my legs, back and core, and to stand tall again, feeling my personal power. I had the energy to reclaim my standing practice and this is where I felt the sense that I could have my own back and take courageous action, embarking on new pursuits in life again.

While these are just my observations, know that there is strong research supporting the effect that movement and posture have on mental health. The antidepressant effects of exercise are well documented[11] and the mantra is *move for mental health, move for your mood, move for a sense of humour*! Any movement will do, it's not only yoga, and it certainly doesn't have to be sport or the gym or even 'exercise'. We're talking a walk around the block, vacuuming, gardening or kitchen discos. If you're curious about posture and mood, tune in to Amy Cuddy's TED talk for an easily digestible discussion of 'power poses'. Erik Peper is a psychologist doing pioneering study into how our posture affects the way we feel. His research shows that the round spine posture we come into when we feel defeated by life, or after spending hours in front of the computer/phone (notice the similarity) lowers subjective mood and energy levels, makes it easier to recall negative memory[12] and it's easier to make someone cry in this shape. Peper also shows that in this curved spine posture we have diminished range of motion for our head to turn and this he postulates makes people feel more threatened and anxious, quite literally because they feel more vulnerable[13]. Conversely, when we stand tall with a long spine and broad chest, with free range of motion to scope the scene around us, we feel safer, more optimistic and energized[14]. There's nothing fluffy about this stuff. Try if for yourself – stand taller, breathe more expansively – and you will feel lighter and brighter.

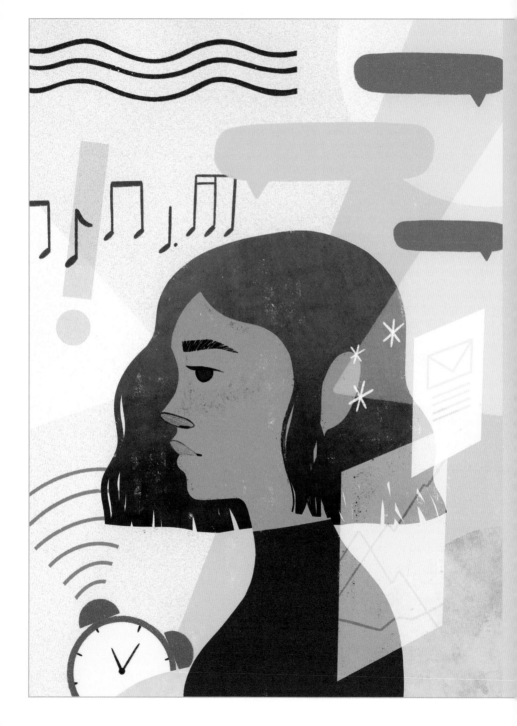

PART ONE

Stress & Burnout

Modern life is fast paced and full on for everyone, and that's before we throw in any curveballs or crises, like illness, conflict or job woes. The catch cry is 'I don't have enough time'. Ask anyone how they're doing and their response is likely to include the word 'busy'. Nine-to-five is genuinely a relic of the past and a side-hustle is becoming the norm. Stress is a modern epidemic. For most of us it's more a case of 'rushing man/woman's syndrome'[15] but at the other end of the spectrum we have diagnoses of acute stress reaction, PTSD and burnout.

WHY ARE WE ALL SO STRESSED?

Let's take a look at the nature of modern life and stress. It's not all doom and gloom – as you read through this next section I hope that reflecting on the sources and signs of stress might also bring to light the antidotes to it. Set the intention to consider ways you can minimize these factors or employ strategies that could provide a protective buffer.

From the moment we wake to the moment our heads hit the pillow, there is a cacophony of sounds – the alarm clock, the pinging notifications from school, work, family and friends, appliances that beep at you until you turn them off, mowers, cars, background music, other people's music, conversation, and our precious downtime filled with screens and more noise.

It is not only sensory overload, but information and choice overload too. We can become experts on just about anything at the click of a button, but let's just hope we've found a reliable source. A quick browse of our supermarket shelves or an online search and you'll see why we can wind up paralysed by the number of options available.

Take one trip on public transport at rush hour and you'll understand why commuters feel squeezed, in mind and body. Blow your nose after a visit to any bustling city and you will see the physical residue of pollution right before you.

Whether you want it or not, we are constantly ambushed by advertising, from product placement, paid partnerships, the plastering of posters all over our public transport, in our newspapers and newsfeeds, on the radio, and where I grew up in Australia, they even wrote it in the sky – literally, using vapour trails, and towing banners from sea planes. All of this fuels a myriad of false needs, perpetuating this nonsense notion that we're simply not enough in ourselves, creating an insatiable hunger to acquire more, do more and be more. When the CEO of a leading pharmaceutical brand can stand up in public and say that they are primarily in the business of keeping shareholders happy, over the business of health care[16], you know as a society we have something troubling to address. One battle at a time though. For you, in the midst of a tough time, please just do your best to shield yourself from this bombardment and see through this artificially manufactured lack. You are already enough, and no shiny object will enhance your happiness or value as a human being.

We are more plugged in and switched on than ever before but also arguably more disconnected than ever before too. The world has become smaller with the advent of social media, making it easier to stay current with others, wherever they are in the world. But as a society there is greater fragmentation and isolation as family units are often flung from one side of the globe to the other, making real hands-on support harder to come by. Comparison fuelled by social media contributes to a feeling of perceived inadequacy, some are plagued by bullies in this new faceless way of interacting and loneliness is common. In addition to our real-world burden there's an online life to manage and algorithms to feed. The ubiquitous nature of technology means that we're seldom ever doing 'nothing' any more. We're glued to our screens on our commute or if we're waiting for a friend, we'll while away that time with scrolling. Got a moment spare? The screen is always there to fill that gap.

As a society we're losing the ability to just 'be', addicted to stimulation and doing. We're stuck in relentless 'productivity' with stillness feeling like an uncomfortable waste of time. Phrases like 'FOMO', 'I'll sleep when I'm dead', 'you snooze you lose' all demonstrate this glorification of busyness. Sleep deprivation is worn like a badge of honour and every time I hear someone quote that Richard Branson only needs four hours of sleep I want to explode. Adult human beings need seven to nine hours of sleep every night to function, to be able to think straight. (If you're not getting that, please don't worry. There will be tips here to help you compensate!)

The point is there is nothing indulgent about getting the sleep you need. There is nothing lazy about resting, especially when good sleep is hard to come by. There is nothing selfish about taking time for restorative practices when you're in the middle of a tough time or healing from one or just being proactive to avoid being bowled over by a future one. We wouldn't celebrate someone for getting by on drinking only a few glasses of water a day, why should our sleep needs be any different?

Life squeezes us from all angles – our environment, our work, our family life and living in uncertain political times.

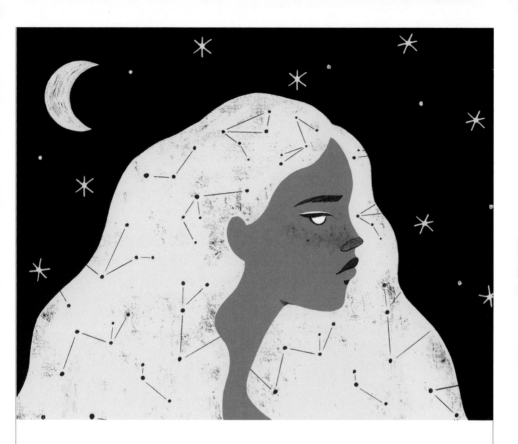

The concerns are real and the mental and emotional loads are huge. Many of us also feel an overwhelming sense of pressure to get ahead, or just to keep up. The reality for most parents is that everyone shares some kind of financial burden and we all have responsibility for tending to the kids. Grandparents are shouldering this burden too. Everyone is doing it all. Our children feel this same competition and pressure to perform from such an early age, with the scheduling of before- and after-school clubs, tutoring, sport, music to fit in, tests to ace, sparkling careers and Instafame to jostle for.

If you're feeling frazzled, it's really no wonder, is it? Drop the guilt, shake off the blame. Life is what it is, but we can go about it differently. It's ok to take a breather. We all need to learn how to slow down. We need to reclaim the ability to relax! We can give ourselves permission to sleep, to rest, to soften into the moment. There will only ever be 24 hours in a day, we just need to look at how we're using that time. Technology and social media have revolutionized our lives and now we need to harness them to our benefit, with mindful usage and remembering to unplug and recharge ourselves just as we're committed to managing our devices. And if this is what we need to do to navigate just the daily grind, then we need to dish out an enormous helping of tenderness and go gently when we're in the crush of life-changing events.

We simply can't afford to be complacent about stress. It has significant ramifications for our health, well-being, relationships, work performance and enjoyment of life itself. Stress has been linked with a host of mental, emotional and physical disorders including depression, anxiety, chest pain, heart attacks, high blood pressure, strokes, obesity, headaches, gastrointestinal conditions, skin problems and insomnia...

BUT it's not all bad!

It's also really helpful to acknowledge that not all stress is negative! The right kind of stress and in the right kind of amounts is the very stuff that keeps us growing as people and engaged in life. Without stress we would become bored very quickly. Stress calls on us to step up and the

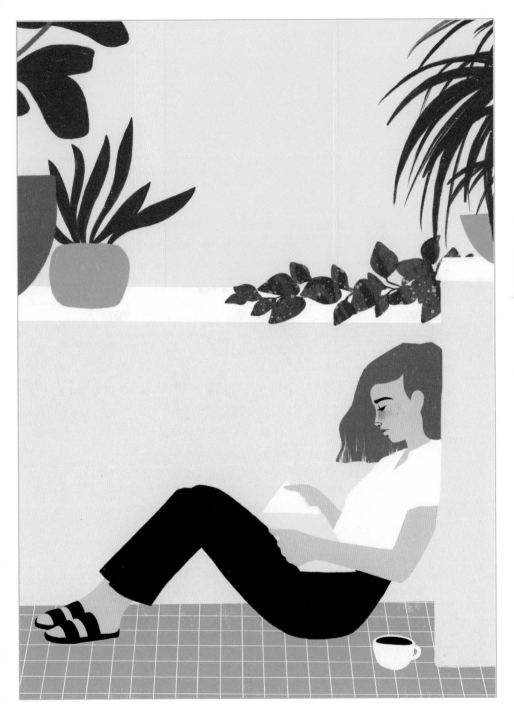

Stress & Burnout

lessons we learn from these experiences can not only boost our resilience and reveal our strengths but also add meaning and purpose to our lives. Look at all the inspiring people out there who have mined their heartache to become incredible agents of change in this world.

Researchers have made a distinction between negative stress, such as relationship breakdown, called 'distress', and positive stress, such as scoring a promotion, stress that is good for us, called 'eustress'[17]. After looking at all the ways we are impinged by stress, let's look at some of the ways stress can be beneficial.

While stress is not only inevitable, it can also be fertile ground for evolution. In fact our attitude toward stress can make all the difference between it harming and helping us. Psychologists have coined a phrase for our relationship with stress, calling it our 'stress mindset'[18]. People who believe that stressful challenges can enhance focus, boost motivation and offer learning opportunities are said to have a positive stress mindset. Conversely, viewing stress as negative, debilitating and unpleasant would constitute a negative stress mindset. Research shows that how you feel about stress can impact on how stress affects you[19] and just reframing how you think about it might provide you with some protective buffer against adversity. Kelly McGonigal says it beautifully: 'while excess stress can take a toll on you, the very things that cause it are often the same things that make life rewarding and full.'[20] Her TED talk 'How to make stress your friend' is a nourishing listen[21]. Let's just plant that seed and perhaps it can be of use to you.

Benefits of stress

- Stress can motivate you, boost your performance and efficiency, and help you meet daily challenges – think of how a deadline propels you into action.

- Short-term stress can boost your brain power. Research suggests there are benefits to your memory, focus and cognitive function[22].

- Short-term stress can boost your immune function[23].

- Stress can boost your resilience.[24] Even crises, in time, can have their silver linings as seen in post-traumatic growth.

- Manageable stress may help protect against oxidative damage, which is linked to ageing and disease[25].

- Stress can enhance bonding[26]. When we see stress as a shared experience it can enhance our feeling of connection. As loved ones turn to each other in times of stress this can strengthen relationships. The outpouring of love and care shown can be deeply affirming.

- Remember that stress is also essential for survival – it's the vital warning system that triggers the fight or flight response, motivating us to take action to keep ourselves safe.

WHAT ACTUALLY IS STRESS?

In its simplest definition, stress is our body's response to challenges from a situation or event. The trigger will vary between individuals but common themes are experiencing something new or unexpected, anything that threatens your safety, feeling a lack of control or when there is an imbalance of resources in relation to the challenge you're facing. When we're faced with a stressor (it was designed to be triggered by sabre tooth tigers, these days our inbox can cause the same internal cascading of stress hormones), the fight or flight response is activated, helping us respond to the perceived danger. As we've already discussed on page 54, if our stress response is triggered repeatedly or stress becomes excessive or chronic, this can be very depleting, making us feel like we're stuck on high alert.

How do we know we're 'stressed'? What does it feel like?

Stress shows up in many different ways and can change over time. We tend to have our own set of symptoms or warning signs and it's empowering to identify how stress personally manifests for you, so you can take swift restorative action.

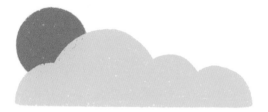

» We feel it in our physical bodies, experienced as pain or tension, increased heart rate, sweaty hands, feeling light-headed or faint, or we might feel jittery and jumpy or lethargic and heavy.

» It can affect our immune system, lowering our defences, illnesses and conditions tend to linger or we go from one ailment to the next.

» We feel it in our guts – bloating, unsettled stomach, digestive complaints.

» It shows up in our mind and our mood with irritability, negativity, worry or overthinking, feeling overwhelmed, difficulty focusing, trouble quietening the mind and forgetfulness.

» It can affect our energy levels, manifesting as fatigue or loss of sexual desire.

» It disturbs our sleep – despite feeling tired, stress interferes with our ability to fall asleep, get back to sleep, the quality of our sleep and can result in early morning waking.

WHAT IS BURNOUT & HOW IS IT DIFFERENT FROM STRESS?

Stress and burnout[27] can look similar and it can be difficult to know where stress ends and burnout begins. Stress is the starting phase of burnout and if the stress is excessive and prolonged, the cumulative effect can be burnout, resulting in a state of emotional, mental and physical exhaustion, feeling completely overwhelmed and unable to cope. It is not possible to have burnout without stress, but it is possible to be stressed without it leading to burnout.

Broadly speaking stress can be conceived as too much happening at once and people who are stressed can imagine feeling better once they've got a handle on the challenges at hand. Burnout can be understood as not enough in the tank to cope, feeling utterly drained, empty and beyond caring. In a state of burnout problems can seem insurmountable and it's difficult to muster up the energy for anything, leaving you feeling increasingly helpless and hopeless. You can wind up feeling like you've got absolutely nothing left to give. From my own experience, I call it 'energetic bankruptcy'; my nervous system felt fried, like I'd been hit by a freight train. The worrying thing is that while people feel very aware of being stressed, we can descend into burnout without noticing initially. The danger is we can get used to feeling highly stressed and on the cusp of burnout and accept it as normal. We need to be vigilant about the early warning signs like disturbed sleep, constant fatigue, difficulty concentrating or unexplained pains and take notice when compensatory behaviours (a reliance on alcohol, sugar and caffeine) creep in.

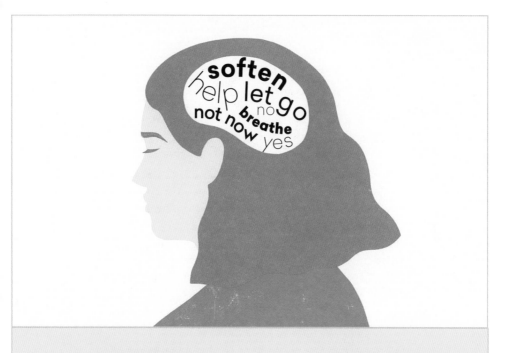

STRESS	BURNOUT
Help! I need an extra day in the week!	**Stop the world, I want to get off.**
Over-engaged or too much effort	Disengaged or able to muster little effort
Reactive or over-reactive emotions	Emotions feel distant, dulled or blunted
Feeling of urgency or hyperactivity	Sense of helplessness and hopelessness
Diminished energy	Diminished motivation or hope
Can lead to anxiety	Can lead to depression
Toll is primarily physical	Toll is primarily emotional

What causes burnout?

Traditionally burnout was viewed in the context of work but anyone is vulnerable to burnout whether the cause is your job or other demands and responsibilities, such as for parents, carers and athletes.

'Work'-related causes of burnout (this is just as relevant in the home)

» Feeling a lack of control: insufficient resources needed to work effectively or an inability to influence decisions that affect you

» Feeling unappreciated, a lack of recognition or reward for good work

» Unclear, unreasonable or unrealistic job expectations

» Monotonous, tedious tasks or work that isn't challenging

» Work that doesn't draw on your strengths and interests

» Operating in a high-pressure, dysfunctional, toxic or chaotic environment

» Conflict between organizational values and personal values

Lifestyle causes of burnout

» Poor work/life balance

» Lack of social support

» Over-committing, taking on too many responsibilities

» Poor sleep, exercise or nutrition habits

» In cases of 'exercise burnout' the two primary causes are overtraining and insufficient recovery time. It's not just athletes, anyone can overdo it

Contributing personality traits

» Perfectionism

» Pessimism

» High-achieving personality types

» Overwhelming need to be in control and difficulty delegating or asking for help

Cultural causes

» Prolific messages encouraging consumerism

» Glorification of busyness and productivity

» Prioritization of profit

How does burnout feel?

Physical signs – tired all the time even when you've met your sleep needs, greater sensitivity to noise, frequent headaches, palpitations, shortness of breath, muscular pain and tension, great difficulty relaxing, supressed immune system and frequent illness, bowel upset, change in appetite, nausea, insomnia.

Emotional signs – feelings of failure, defeat, detachment and loneliness, loss of motivation and hope, numbing or diminished enjoyment and sense of satisfaction. Feeling like you are not your 'normal self'. Feeling teary, reactive, irritable, angry, cynical and a sense of apathy.

Mental signs – indecision, poor concentration and memory, hard to switch off, feeling wired, mind fog, feeling overloaded, anxiety, depression, paranoia.

The Maslach Burnout Inventory[28], designed to measure burnout, can help you get clear on where you are at and please reach out to your doctor for support.

What do we need to prioritize during times of stress and burnout? How do we heal? How do we protect ourselves from future stress? Look at the Vitality Wheel diagram on page 70, annotated with lifestyle choices and habits. We will develop each of these with the practices that follow.

The skills key to navigating stress and burnout

Mindfulness – building the ability to notice what is happening within you, your warning signs, what is unfolding outside of you, and managing your response. Developing the skill of checking in and taking swift recuperative action.

Connection with your body – noticing how your body feels, building a language for sensation, hearing messages from your body. Also cultivating tenderness toward your body.

The ability to relax – understanding the difference between tension and relaxation and being able consciously to release physical tension.

Energy management – the ability to notice your energy levels, to re-energize and lift your mood.

Breathing – reclaiming the ability to breathe naturally and expansively, helping you come home to yourself, to be your own safe place.

THE ANTIDOTES TO STRESS & BURNOUT – WHAT YOU CAN DO

SLEEP, REST, RELAXATION & BREATHING – make them a priority and appreciate their value! Building a toolkit of restorative practices and time to enjoy an absence of stimulation. Greater understanding of when to push and when to surrender.

VALUES & PURPOSE – what matters most to you? Understanding causes of your stress/burnout.

GOALS – the intention is to soothe and relax, to replenish and restore, less striving!

MOOD BOOSTERS – gratitude, kindness, learning how to calm yourself, time- and energy-efficient mood alchemy like scent and colour.

MOVEMENT & NUTRITION – move for mental health and keep it soft and restorative, not vigorous or depleting. Nourish your mood by eating for stress or burnout and utilize simple strategies like organization and planning.

COPING SKILLS – stress mindset, growth mindset, boundaries of control, healthy tech use.

PHYSICAL ENVIRONMENT – get outside and prioritize making your home environment harmonious.

SOCIAL CONNECTION – who's in your corner, asking for help and shaping how it is given, tailoring the nature of social interaction according to your energy levels.

Create a spot in your home that can be your haven of calm.

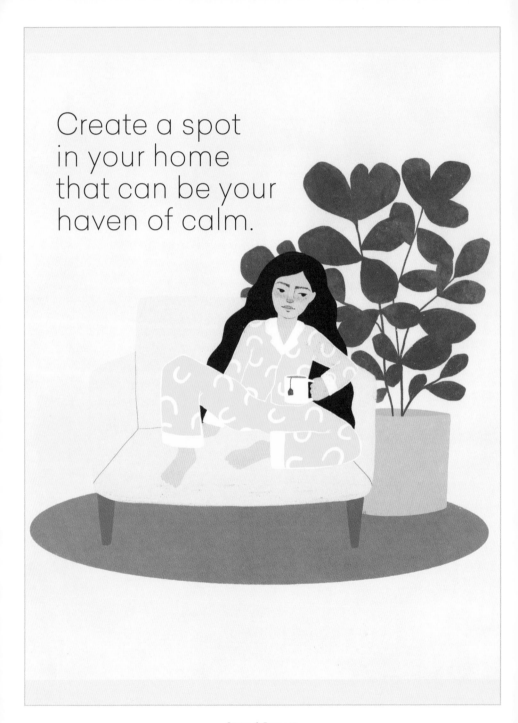

THE PRACTICES FOR STRESS & BURNOUT

Effortless recharge

When we're stressed, exhausted or burned out, we need strategies to help us effortlessly receive energy. Build a toolkit of ways you can receive this transfusion of light and life. Here are some suggestions:

Draw on nature's healing properties – when energy is low, turn to Mother Nature to reinvigorate you. Can you gaze on the beauty of a flower to cultivate a sense of awe? Can you imbibe the warmth of the sun on your skin or take in a sunset? Can you watch the moving cloudscape and remember how swiftly things change? Let the breeze blow away stagnant energy and release anything else you no longer need. Allow the rain to cleanse and wash away what's done.

Turn to your inside environment for comfort – this is not about living in a show home, but channelling a sense of 'outer order creates inner harmony'. A little tidying or cleaning can genuinely pave the way for greater clarity of thought. Create a spot in your home that can be your haven of calm. It could be a sunny nook, an armchair, your bed dressed with linen you love. Dot around your home little focal points that lift you up: a pot plant by your bed, a cushion or throw on your sofa that you love the colour or texture of, a photograph by the kitchen sink to gaze on while you tend to the dishes, or a vase with a cut stem on the dining table. Spritz some room spray or light a scented candle to create a nurturing ambiance. Nothing fancy required, just something to anchor your attention, bringing you peace.

Nourishing resource library – build a library of podcasts, TED talks, audio books, music, guided relaxations or yoga nidra, a form of guided relaxation. When you're feeling depleted let these resources uplift and empower you.

 Planting a seed: Do you notice that your problems seem more manageable or do you feel more resourceful in response to them when you have topped up your energy bank? What are some other ways you can fill yourself up?

Spritz some room spray or light a scented candle to create a nurturing ambiance.

Relaxation

It's not pointless, lazy or just 'nice to have'. Here's why it's essential:

» Slowing down allows us to get in synch with our natural rhythms, so we can hear messages from the body, like hunger, weariness or anxiety. Awareness of these cues means we can take targeted action and bring ourselves back to balance with less disruption

» Relaxation promotes healing, detoxification and cellular repair, strengthening the immune system and soothing the nervous system. If you don't find time to rest and replenish, your body is likely to find it for you, most often at the least opportune moment via enforced rest due to illness or injury

» Time out provides us with the opportunity for reflection, encouraging creativity

» Relaxation practices like mindfulness change the structure of the brain[29], boosting resilience and mental health

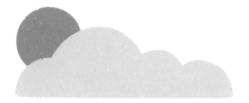

What is relaxation?

Relaxation is a state of calm, ease, harmony and peacefulness, with a softening, expansive quality. Knowing the opposite to relaxation helps clarify what it's all about – an absence of effort, tension, ambition, striving and conflict.

Learning how to relax

Relaxation is the antidote to stress, in fact it's impossible to be relaxed and stressed at the same time, given they activate opposing branches of your nervous system. To reclaim the ability to let go, first we must learn the difference between tension and relaxation. We're seldom aware of just how much tension we hold in the body and if you're not aware of it, it's very hard to release it. Even when we're acutely aware of tight spots it can be hard to know how to create softening. Some gentle physical exertion will help you let go more effortlessly. It's easy to equate relaxation with 'doing nothing' – stillness is just one way but there are many gentle moving practices that can be just as effective. The following sequence connects you with your core, helping you strengthen without requiring much energy and then relax without even thinking about it.

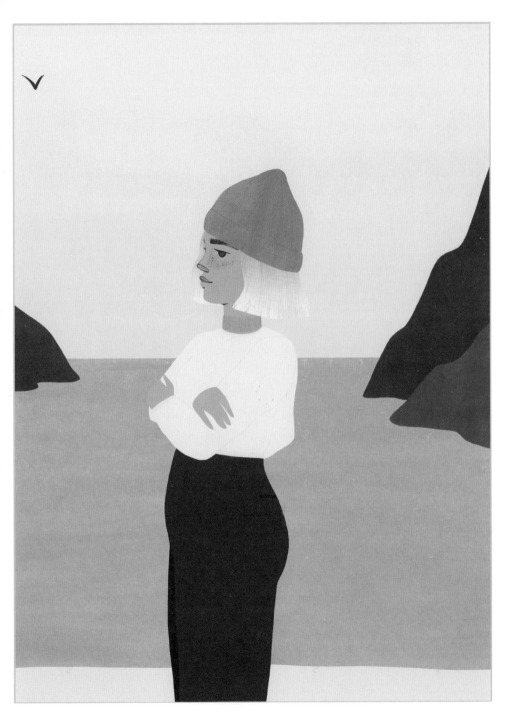

Stress & Burnout

Core connection

Lie down on your back with your knees bent and your feet flat on the floor. Notice how it feels to be lying here, relaxing your whole body as best you can. It's ok if there is some resistance to being still and if your mind is darting about away from the present moment. Bring your attention to your hands and your feet. Place your palms flat on your thighs. As you breathe in, let your body relax, enjoying that there is nothing to be done. As you breathe out, press your feet firmly into the floor and your hands down onto your thighs, feeling the muscles this activates in your arms, chest, stomach and thighs. You might be surprised how much your stomach muscles leap into action. Just notice their engagement via the action of your hands and feet, don't try to tense them. Take the whole inhalation to soften and let go of this work and the whole out breath to press your hands and feet down firmly. After ten repetitions, let your arms fall where comfortable and allow your knees to drop toward each other. Notice how much easier it is to relax now and how your mind is more securely focused on the present moment. Check in and see if your rate of breathing feels any different from when you began. Maybe it is a little slower now.

Next, bring your arms down by your sides with your palms facing downwards, in preparation for the Dynamic Bridge. As you breathe in, raise your arms overhead to the floor behind you. As you breathe out, lower your arms back down by your sides and raise your hips and chest as high as you can. Inhale to lower your hips and raise

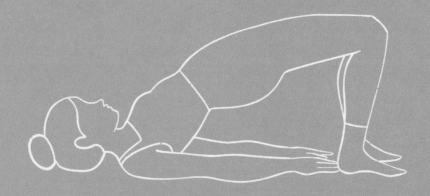

your arms, exhale to lower your arms and raise your hips. Repeat this ten times, feeling the engagement of your buttocks and thighs and the powerful stretch for the front of your body as you lift into the bridge. Once complete, notice the energy circulating in your legs, hips, abdomen and lower back. Feel the breath as it moves through your abdomen – perhaps it feels more spacious there now? Notice if there is a relationship between the quality of your breathing and the quality of your mind.

Lastly, having gently worked your body and focused your mind, come to rest in stillness in Butterfly pose. Place a pillow beneath your head, bend your knees and bring the soles of your feet together, allowing your knees to descend toward the floor, supporting them with cushions for extra comfort. Drape an eye pillow over your eyes to block out light and add to the sense of being held. Feel the earth rise to meet you and allow your whole body to be held. Let your hands rest on your tummy, feeling them move with your breath. In your belly lies a deep reservoir of kindness and calm. Let your mind's eye rest there and stay as long as you feel comfortable – ten breaths or ten minutes.

 Planting a seed: With regular practice of this sequence, notice if you become more aware of tension creeping into your body throughout your day. As that mindfulness grows, notice if you also become more skilled in listening to your body, learning what it needs to let go. Your body will tell you what to do. In time, this may help you move through your day with greater peace and ease, even in the face of difficult moments.

Hand sequence

Try this hand yoga sequence at your desk, the kitchen sink or while sitting on the sofa. Use it to bring circulation and feeling back into your fingers, hands and limbs and to experience a sense of calm. Clasp your hands with the right on top and squeeze them together for a moment. Change, clasping your hands with the left on top and hold for a moment. With a moderate pace, alternate this squeezing action ten times. Then shake out your hands and feel the energy circulating around them. Next interlace your fingers and squeeze your hands firmly together. Unlace your fingers then interlace your hands again with the other thumb on top. Again, with a moderate pace, alternate the interlace and squeeze ten times. Stretch your arms out in front of you, palms facing each other. Take your right arm on top of your left, now turn your thumbs to point downwards and interlace your fingers. Draw your hands toward you and through, as far as comfortable without losing the interlacing of your fingers, repeating this movement toward you and away six times. Repeat the sequence with your left arm on top. Cup your hands in your lap and feel the buzz of energy. Enjoy sitting in stillness feeling this warmth and enjoying the absence of effort.

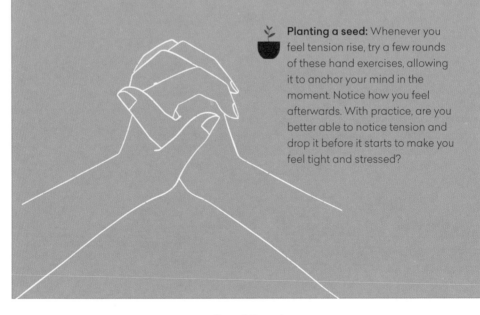

Planting a seed: Whenever you feel tension rise, try a few rounds of these hand exercises, allowing it to anchor your mind in the moment. Notice how you feel afterwards. With practice, are you better able to notice tension and drop it before it starts to make you feel tight and stressed?

Slow down

We are often on autopilot, zooming through our day at breakneck speed. Slow down, soften into everyday actions and you might notice this changes the quality of your whole day. There is a false economy of hurry, haste and speed. When we take care, we are more effective and we're more likely to get the job done right, first time. Start small by imbuing these actions with presence: how you apply your moisturiser or brush your teeth, how you eat – even a few savoured mouthfuls will do, a mindful shower, how you fold the washing or unstack the dishwasher. Parents, here's one not for the faint-hearted...try slowing down to walk at your child's pace. Inevitably, your inner voice will tell you 'I don't have time for this' and the stress hormones cascade. Every time it does, replace it with the affirmation '*I have all the time I need*'. Even if you don't believe it, it's a useful distraction from the former statement.

 Planting a seed: Notice when you're speeding up or when you're making mistakes. Take a long breath out and commit to slowing down. Remind yourself you might only have to do it once when you do it with care. Do you notice more incidental joyful moments when you take your time?

The mindful check in

Build the habit of checking in with yourself, head, heart and body, at different intervals in your day. It could be first thing in the morning, as you hop into the car or after the school run, as you sit down at your desk, before you take a lunch break, when the 2pm energy slump hits, after dinner, or before bed. The ability to notice where you're at forms the foundation for self-care. The mindful check in is an opportunity to observe your inner cues like hunger, fatigue, tension or pain, your ability to focus or concentrate, feelings of loneliness or desire to be alone, or the presence of any emotion. Observe without judgement or criticism for a minute or less if you're time squeezed, setting the intention to lovingly tend to any needs you find.

 Planting a seed: As you build this practice, what do you learn about yourself – the causes of your stress or burnout, and your warning signs? Over time, can you spot them sooner, take more proactive action and feel more in control?

Come home to your body

To deepen your awareness of your physical body, having a broad vocabulary of physical sensations will help. Ponder these words a while and refer to this list while you are engaging in a mindful check in or during your yoga:

Sharp, dull, radiating, pulsing, shooting, throbbing, fizzing, pins and needles, warm, cold, tight, loose, stringy, achy, heavy, light, constricted, loose, open, spacious, expansive, faint, goosebump, fluid, stuck, frozen, numb, zingy, floppy, puffy, jittery, fuzzy, twitchy, shivers, tingling, trembling, dense, faint, dizzy, bloated, smooth, soft, energized.

Where do you notice these sensations and do they change with time? Is there some kind of message in them? Are they suggesting to you any kind of movement in response? There is no right or wrong, just let curiosity guide you.

 Planting a seed: As your vocab for sensation grows do you feel a greater awareness of your body? Does this help you befriend your body and boost your motivation to be tender and kind toward it?

A ritual to rest your senses

The antidote to all the sensory overload in your day: run a bath and set the intention to restore your energy. This is not an opportunity to run through your 'to do' list, this is a chance to enjoy an absence of effort and stimulation. Let others know that you do not wish to be disturbed and if you have kids, allocate responsibility elsewhere so you have complete permission and freedom to detach.

Add to the water some magnesium flakes for their anti-inflammatory properties, some lavender for its soothing scent or Epsom salts to deepen muscular relaxation. As you soak, visualize tension leaving your body, burdens being dropped and held by the water instead. Enjoy submerging your ears beneath the water and notice the profound quiet. Close your eyes and rest your senses. There is nothing to achieve here, just a letting go. If you're feeling sleepy only stay here a while, then rest your head against the bath and maintain an awareness of your body softening and being warmed and supported by the water. We don't want to fall asleep here, keep tethering your mind to the sensation of your body relaxing. If your mind wanders, use a mantra to keep it anchored on something constructive. Try *'the world can wait'* or *'there is nothing required of me right now'*.

A little caveat with this exercise: our addiction to busyness and our state of high alert can make relaxation not only feel foreign but also uncomfortable. Relentless doing distracts us from our thoughts and feelings, so when we stop we're faced with these inner experiences and it can feel overwhelming. If this resonates, go gently. In fact there is some telling research that shows you're not alone…in 11 studies participants were found to prefer self-administering electric shocks rather than being left alone with their thoughts, suggesting that many of us prefer to be doing something, rather than nothing, even when that something is negative[30]. If relaxing in stillness feels confronting, come back to this practice and use others that bring your focus onto movement or nature.

 Planting a seed: Set the intention to notice moments through your day where there's an absence of effort, really drinking in moments of peace. You also might like to observe how you are held and supported in life – the chair beneath you, the bed that cradles you, the earth beneath your feet or the loving arms that wrap you up in a warm embrace. Allow yourself to feel this visceral sense of being comforted and cared for.

The healing power of breathing

How we breathe has a powerful impact on how we feel. When we're stressed the breath tends to get caught up in the chest, feeling short and tight. When we allow the breath to be slower, more expansive and down in the abdomen, it helps us feel calmer. There is nothing 'woo woo' about it. Calm, relaxed breathing stimulates the ventral vagal complex, activating the parasympathetic nervous system and its 'rest and digest' response. When we breathe better we're naturally more empathetic, resourceful and resilient in the face of stress, because this way of breathing helps keep the social engagement system online with more blood being directed to parts of the brain responsible for problem-solving, rather than invoking the fight or flight response where blood rushes to the extremities to prepare us for action. Focusing on your breath can be a powerful way to stay anchored in the present moment and a compelling distraction from unhelpful thoughts. Breathe better, feel better.

Breath basics – using movement

Moving with the breath is the easiest way to begin. Rather than trying to breathe in a certain way, focus your mind on movement paired with the breath. You may have experienced that trying to breathe deeply when you are anxious or stressed can amplify your agitation. The solution is moving in time with the inhalation and exhalation.

Lie down with your legs outstretched and your arms down by your sides. For a few moments, just notice how it feels to be lying on the floor, allowing your breath to be exactly as it is. Notice its rhythm, where you feel it move in your body and any qualities like smooth, jerky, even, irregular, short, shallow, deep, tight, expansive, effortless, laboured, loud or quiet. Think of this as establishing your baseline and we'll see what changes naturally arise.

As you breathe in next, raise your arms up toward the ceiling and overhead to the floor behind you, pointing your toes at the same time. Notice a pause at the end of your inhalation. As you breathe out, lower your arms back down by your sides and flex your heels. Notice a pause at the end of your out breath. Match the movement to the comfortable length of your breath (i.e. you don't want to be moving if you've run out of breath, just move faster to be in time with your natural breathing). This doesn't have to be super slow, just make sure it feels comfortable, repeating this arm movement with your breathing ten times. Notice how the movement of the arms helps you take a deeper in breath, making space between the ribs, and as you exhale, the downward movement of the arms creates a bellows-like feeling, igniting the diaphragm to help you more completely empty the lungs. Keep focusing on the movement and allowing it effortlessly to help you breathe more expansively.

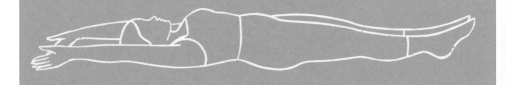

You might observe that the front of your body gets a lovely stretch on the in breath and the back of your body elongates on the out breath. Take the opportunity to enjoy these sensations. Now allow your body to come back to stillness and feel your breathing again. Has it changed from how it felt before – its rhythm, location or quality? Do you notice any other impact such as your energy level, your focus, on the nature of your thoughts? As you become more practiced at this exercise you might like to add a mantra to the movement. On your inhalation repeat the words internally: '*I receive*'. On your exhalation repeat the words: '*I release*'.

 Planting a seed: Throughout your day take a moment to feel your breathing. This isn't thinking about the breath, or changing it consciously, just notice the sensations. By just observing the breath, it begins to regulate itself, smoothing itself out. Start by practising in moments of ease and build to using this tool is times of challenge. What difference does your breathing make in those stressful times?

Breath basics – using sound

Another way to cultivate a feeling of calm is using 'bee breath', similar to a humming sound. Research has shown this can be even more effective in reducing stress than just witnessing the breath or thoughts alone, the longer exhalation and vibration potentially adding to the soothing effect, providing another object on which to anchor the mind[31]. Sit tall, relax your shoulders and take a couple of natural breaths. If it feels good to you, close your eyes. Begin bee breath by keeping your lips closed, breathing in through the nose and exhaling making the sound 'mmm' like a bee. Repeating this, inhaling as needed and humming on the exhalation, for a few minutes or as long as it feels good to you. You might find just a few rounds can cultivate a deeper appreciation or readiness for silence.

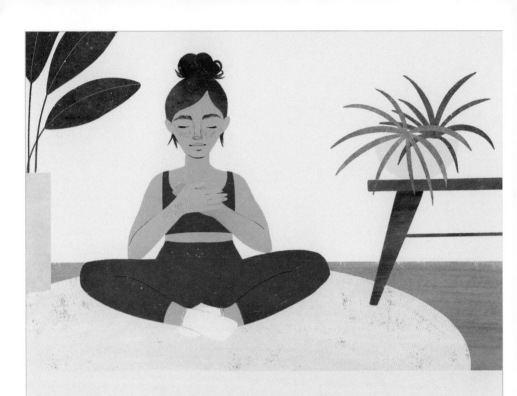

By just observing the breath, it begins to regulate itself, smoothing itself out. Start by practising in moments of ease and build to using this tool is times of challenge.

A ritual of soothing touch

Touch, whether received from another or self-administered, releases oxytocin. Oxytocin is a stress-coping hormone, critical to a sense of feeling safe. It facilitates social bonds, love and belonging, resilience and stress buffering, allowing the body to adapt and heal in response to stress. Drawing on the power of touch, this face, head, neck and shoulder massage has a deeply restorative effect.

Check in and notice how you feel before trying this practice, observing your breathing, your levels of tension, the quality of your mind, and your mood. Engage in the practice or just part of it and note down any changes in how you feel afterwards.

Shoulder rub – take your right hand across your left shoulder beside your neck, press your fingertips in and draw them across the ridge of your shoulder. Repeat this six times, moving further away from your neck with each repetition. Repeat on the other side.

Head turns – relaxing your arms by your sides and your shoulders away from your ears, keeping your chin parallel to the ground, look to the right, then look to your left. Do this three times each way, lubricating the neck.

Shoulder roll – take your fingertips onto your shoulders. As you breathe in bring your elbows forward and upwards and as you exhale, take them back and down, six times. Feel how this frees your chest and shoulders and lifts you into a more upright posture.

Collar bone hang – bring your chin down toward your chest. Starting at the inner tip of your collarbones, press your fingers firmly into the ridge, as if you are hanging from your collarbones by your fingertips. Maintain this pressure while you lift your chin up, stretching your throat. Repeat twice more, moving your hands slightly further apart each time.

Jaw massage – with the first three fingertips of both hands, slide them from the top of your jaw, just below your temples, downwards. Repeat this firmly and slowly three times, allowing your mouth to open as you do so.

Ear pull and rub – hold onto your earlobes and draw them straight down, three times. With your first two fingers, start at your temples, work your way up, over and behind your ear and massage downwards, three times.

Eye socket press – take the pads of your fingers onto your cheek bones and press firmly. Work gradually along them toward your ears. Feel the fresh blood this brings to your face and the tension it releases. If it feels good, return to the spot below of the middle of your eye and finish here with one more sustained press.

Temporal press – bring your thumbs onto your temples and place your fingertips onto your forehead. Imagine you have two goaty horns on your forehead; this is the spot to place your fingertips – you'll feel there is a slight bony ridge there. Gentle pressure here resets the nervous system and relieves tension. If you think of the natural gesture we make when we get bad news – back of the hand to the forehead

– you'll see we are hardwired to restore using these pressure points. Maintain the temporal press for six relaxed breaths and feel how this calms the stress response.

Cup your face – rest your chin in hands and wrap your fingertips up to your temples. Hold here for six calm breaths.

Bathe your eyes – rub your hands together to create warmth, then cup your palms over your eyes, extending tenderness toward yourself for six breaths.

Scalp massage – to refresh your mind, bring your fingertips to your hairline at the centre of your forehead and run them firmly along your scalp, back and down to the nape of your neck. Repeat several times, moving your hands wider apart until you reach your ears and then finish with several strokes of the back of your head and up to your crown, beginning at the base of your skull and taking the hands wider apart until you reach the ears. Feel the resurgence of energy this brings.

Complete this ritual of soothing touch by bringing your hands to your heart and repeating the mantra: '*I feel my breath come home*'. Linger here for at least six smooth, replenishing breaths.

 Planting a seed: Look for opportunities to use elements of this sequence throughout your day. It needn't be in entirety, just one might be enough to soothe you. Jot down moments when this tool might come in handy – this acts as a useful primer to help you remember in the moment. Set the intention to notice stress levels, to respond with compassion, and use any one of these tools to relieve overwhelm.

Mindful tech use

We spend a significant proportion of our waking hours in front of screens, and what we watch, listen to and read has a huge impact on our stress levels. Take stock of how you're using technology and make sure it's serving you:

Think about what you need – observe how you feel before you check in. Will using this technology meet your need?

Be conscious of your tech use – purposefully choose how you plug in.

Be aware – observe how you feel while you're online and afterwards. Check in with the quality of your mind, how your body feels, your mood and your energy. Does it affect how you feel about yourself?

Be selective – relish a social media cull of any accounts that set up the comparison trap, delete apps that don't benefit you. Take a cold, hard look at the figures and see how much time you spend on your apps.

Remove your phone – notice how you feel when your phone is in sight. Even just seeing it can reduce your brainpower[32]. Is the urge to check in irresistible? Screen addiction is real, with our smartphone apps activating the same dopamine-driven neural pathways as slot machines and cocaine[33]. Switching it off or placing it face down isn't enough, make the choice to leave your phone in another room to take a more effective break, especially when your attention is required elsewhere. Make use of silent mode where appropriate and switch off

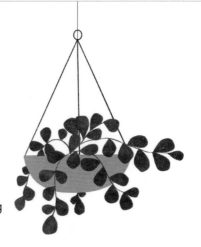

notifications that have you leaping into action unnecessarily.

Keep your tech usage healthy – brainstorm boundaries that you can impose: how often, for what purpose, for how long?

 Planting a seed: Make a concerted effort to bring mindfulness to your tech use and be honest about the impact it has on your well-being. Notice any relationship between the impulse to pick up your phone and stress/anxiety.

Screen addiction is real, with our smartphone apps activating the same dopamine-driven neural pathways as slot machines and cocaine.

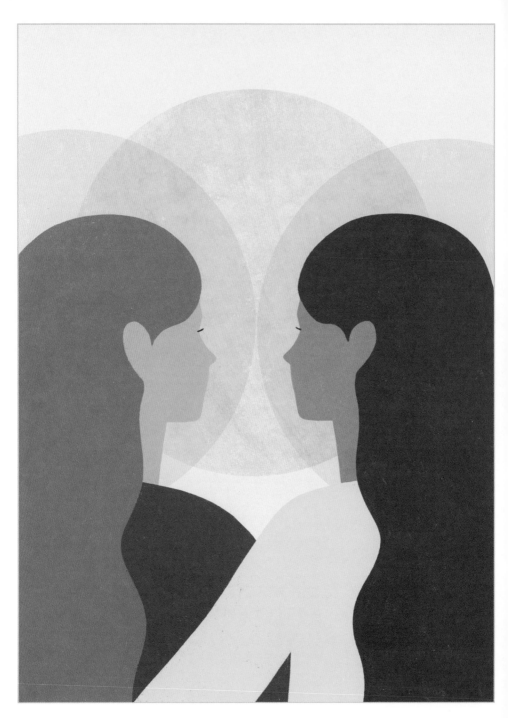

Stress & Burnout

Connection

Human beings are social animals and we need a sense of belonging as much as we need nutritious food and adequate sleep. This web of support is even more critical during times of crisis. We all know we need other people to lift us up but what if our usual means of connection feel inaccessible or too depleting? In tough times, please think about the nature of your social connection and tailor it to your needs and energy levels right now. Give yourself permission to do things differently at this time, rather than withdrawing because it all feels too much. Think about all the people who are in your corner, willing you on. Sometimes we hesitate to reach out, feeling it's not ok to ask for help. Sometimes help is offered and it's not what we need. Give yourself permission not only to ask for help but to shape how help is given. Think about how you've felt in the past toward a friend having a tough time. I'm sure you were just waiting to lend a hand, often not knowing how best to be of support. You actually do people a great service by reaching out for help – it feels good being helpful and it deepens your bonds! It's also important to consider that not everyone will be able to give you the kind of help you need (it's not a lack of love!), so choose wisely and draw on the strengths of the people around you. If you need a kind ear, turn to the person who loves giving that, not the problem solver who specializes in brainstorming a list of things you could do. Different people in different moments will help you through. Let people in as you feel appropriate, knowing that you can shape the following variables:

Who you spend time with – it is ok to opt for company that uplifts and energizes you and to minimize time with people who drag you down. It's not forever. Do what you need to do right now to get by. It's not about putting people in the friend bin. If meeting for conversation feels exhausting, you can change how you interact – see a film together instead. If meeting up as a family feels taxing, ask to get together just the two of you.

Where you come together – You might find that some usual meeting places feel too noisy or crowded right now, so choose an environment that you find replenishing.

What you do during that time – let your friends and family know what you need. There will be people chomping at the bit to show they care. Sometimes it's a kind ear, a hug or some light relief. If you want to talk about it, let them know. Equally, if you don't want to talk about it, let them know you'd prefer some distraction.

When you connect – listen to your energy levels and honour your needs. If going out at night doesn't work for you, perhaps a phone call might be a good alternative. Observe your daily energy rhythms and seek connection when energy allows.

How long you are together – tune in to how you are feeling and allow yourself to dip in and out of connection. Our interactions needn't be long, sometimes all we need is a short and sweet opportunity to connect. If time doesn't allow in-person connection, write a note, leave a voicemail or send a picture, just check in and communicate need or care. Even hearing a loved one's voice can elicit the same stress-busting effect as a warm hug.[34] We often think of letters as a lovely way to document feelings – research shows us that recording a love note could be a beautiful gift and one that keeps on giving.

Even just *imagining* the presence of a loved one can be a buffer against effects of stress[35]. Make a list of all the people on your team and in tough moments, imagine them with you, wrapping you up in their love, whether they are here in earthly form or not.

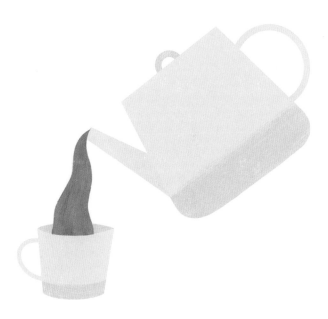

Eating for stress and burnout

We all know what constitutes healthy eating; what's more pressing in tough times is making healthy choices accessible. It's not about labouring in the kitchen, unless you are truly energized by the art of cooking, it's about making nutritious food a priority, planning and organization. The key message here is if you want to think straight, you have to feed your brain. Often, we associate eating with fuelling the body, but 'hanger' is real. We need to eat as much for our mental health and mood. If healthy eating isn't already a habit, when stress levels are high, it's not the time for bold, sweeping changes. We need to keep it as simple as possible and make sure there is decent brain food on the table (and in the freezer). Think along the lines of these nutrient-rich foods that require little preparation or skill: whole grains (you can pop frozen wholemeal pitta bread in the toaster for a warming snack with hummus), eggs, salmon, avocado on oat cakes or your morning toast, lamb, chicken, greens like asparagus that you can pop in foil and cook in the oven, frozen peas, baked beans, edamame beans, bananas, nuts and seeds, or yoghurt. Make sure healthy options are in the house and if you do muster the energy to cook, try to cook in batches that can keep sustaining you.

We're aiming for whole, fresh, colourful, unprocessed foods as much as possible and reducing or eliminating stimulants like sugar, caffeine, alcohol (be brutally honest with yourself about how these things affect your ability to cope and heal). Swap coffee for herbal teas and switch cola, fizzy drinks and alcohol for sparkling water with a pipette of flower essence, like Bach flower

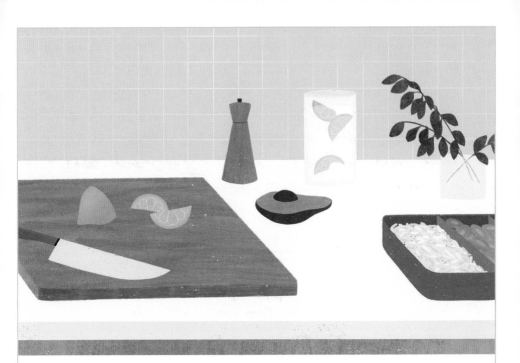

remedy. How you eat has an impact too. Give yourself time for mechanical digestion by properly chewing your food. Eating slowly and mindfully will not only improve digestion and offer you the chance to savour something pleasurable but you're also more likely to notice feelings of fullness and satisfaction.

 Planting a seed: Get to know yourself. Be honest about what works and doesn't work for you and take action. Make sure the healthiest option is the easiest one and keep your home well stocked. When energy, clarity or mood flag, ask yourself when was the last time you imbibed a tall glass of water or ate something life-giving.

Move for mental health

Research shows that all types of movement can be beneficial for stress management[36]. How that looks for each individual will be different and the key to choosing the right exercise for you right now depends on what you find intrinsically enjoyable and where you're placed on the stress–burnout continuum. You may find that movement you typically enjoy is too depleting, even stress-inducing, if you are in a state of burnout. Any movement can help relieve stress – cardio, resistance training, meditative/creative pursuits like yoga, Pilates, tai chi or dance, or everyday activities like vacuuming or gardening. The general guidelines are 150 minutes per week of moderate-intensity aerobic exercise. Leave the vigorous stuff for another time unless it's genuinely cathartic for you. Walking in nature's beauty is a perfect stress buster, or consider swimming because the water can help you feel supported. Keep it varied and light-hearted – no gruelling or punishing workouts, move with a friend, move with music, take lots of breaks or exercise for short durations spaced out through your day. And when you're running on empty, lie down on the floor and turn to your soothing stretches for restorative movement – this definitely counts.

 Planting a seed: Notice the impact that movement has on your energy, mood and mental clarity. If you feel a dip, what movement could you turn to as a pick-me-up? Our needs are constantly changing so make sure you are taking a compassionate and responsible approach to movement, with choices that reflect where you are today.

Mindsets

Your perception of stress itself

We talked earlier about 'stress mindset', how our attitude to stress makes a difference to how it affects us. As best you can, see if you can adopt an open-minded view about stress. Rather than focusing on all the potential harm stress can cause, the ways we can fail or how life could go wrong, focus your mind on the different ways you can grow and learn in response to this tough time. We will look at post-traumatic growth in greater detail in the change section. Sometimes the healing passage of time is necessary before we can begin to entertain the thought of silver linings, but it is worth planting the seed here.

You have every right to have a human response to your own challenge and the sources of your tough time need to be validated.

Your perception of *your* stress

Don't compare your stress to the struggle of others, unless it helps you out of a self-pity party. Even two people in the midst of the same kind of event may have a totally different experience – perhaps this is their first real experience of illness or loss, or maybe this is a trigger to a previous event. There are a whole host of variables at play. Someone else may be facing far greater challenges but this does not diminish your burden. You have every right to have a human response to your own challenge and the sources of your tough time need to be validated. By all means, give thanks for your blessings but don't negate your own feelings and needs because it doesn't serve you, or anyone else. Don't compare how you think you are coping to how others *appear* to be coping either. What we see is just the tip of an iceberg. A healthy dose of compassion all round is more helpful. Comparing yourself now to how you were before life got tough seldom helps. How you are feeling right now will change, go gently on yourself and give yourself time to reclaim your sparkle.

Growth mindset, mistakes and perfectionism

Cultivating a growth mindset, making peace with imperfection (hello, you're human too) and embracing mistakes can help difficult experiences roll from our shoulders with greater ease. Growth mindset, a phrase coined by Carol Dweck[37], is the understanding that abilities and intelligence can be developed, as opposed to a fixed mindset which assumes that our intelligence, strengths and creative abilities are fixed or what you're born with.

Developing a growth mindset helps you reframe challenges, failure and setbacks as learning opportunities rather than seeing them as confirmation of lack. Science shows that you can teach an old dog new tricks as evidenced by neuroplasticity[38] and that forms the basis of this whole book – there are skills that you can learn that will help you cope and heal. Our efforts do make a difference, we can exert control and we can grow and evolve our whole lives long. Turn 'I can't' into 'I am learning to...' There is great power in the word 'yet'. It is coming. Hang in there.

Your attitude to mistakes and perfectionism will have an impact on your stress levels too. Don't harangue yourself for boo-boos, we all make them, what's done is done. Instead, swiftly make any necessary reparations, including self-forgiveness. You can do a bad thing but that doesn't necessarily make you a bad person. Guilt motivates us to adhere to our moral compass, shame often propels us into self-defence. Ask yourself what did that experience teach you and what might you do differently next time? Mistakes are another opportunity to step up and develop grit. If you feel paralysed by rigid ideals on your performance, ask yourself if 'done to a lower standard' is preferable to 'excellent but incomplete'. Consider how sustainable this ideal is – life, we hope, will be a marathon and not a sprint. Bear in mind you are just one person, your resources are finite, there are only 24 hours in a day and this is just one task or role of many. Adjust your expectations accordingly, *prioritize* and take values-led action. Learn to sit with the discomfort of incompletions and relish declaring an end to your day. Down tools and take that long cathartic sigh out. It's not time for work now, it *can* wait! Now it's time to tend to your energy bank.

Make a life map

In turbulent times breaking life down into different areas can help us get a handle on things, and the act of acknowledging the areas of life that are going well can better ground us. It's very easy to fall into the trap of thinking everything has gone to pot when really it's one or two areas of life affected. There may be times when it genuinely feels like everything is spiralling out of control and we need to remind ourselves that it won't be like this forever. The task at hand, then, is to keep our energy bank topped up as best we can, seek out support and chip away at the source of our stress, if that's possible. Making a life map can help us define a boundary to our burden, and work out where to place our energy and attention.

This exercise is a visual tool and you can get as creative as you like with it. Seek out a large piece of paper and use pencil or pen to map out different areas of your life that are important to you. This will be different for everyone, but some suggestions might be family, love or relationships, work, study, personal growth, leisure, learning, social connection, household, community, health, downtime, finances and spirituality. Represent these however you like with text or shapes, use colour and highlight the things that require your attention. Jot down worries or fears if you like. Observe the areas of life in which you're functioning well, express a feeling of thankfulness and give yourself a pat on the back for your accomplishments there. Identify where your sources of stress or burnout lie and mark these on your map, bringing them to the light. Look over your map and if there are problems that don't belong to you, or worries that you can drop, relish crossing these out.

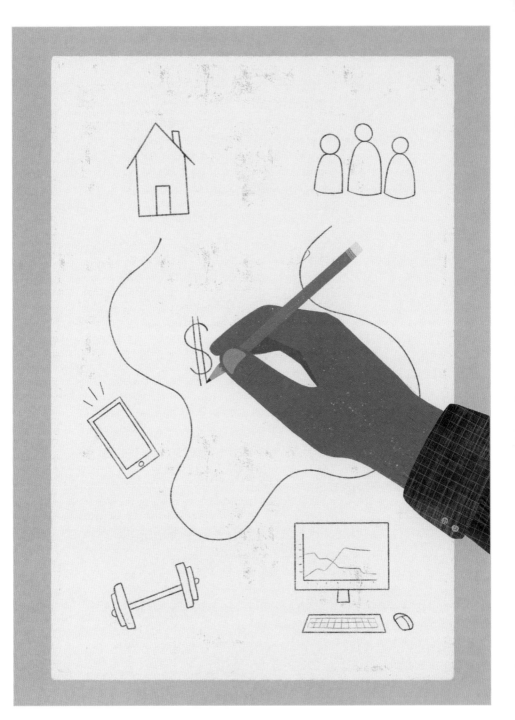

They do not need to drain you of your time and energy. Of the things on your map that do need attention the vital question then becomes: *can I do anything about this*? This question of what's in our control guides us in our action plan.

Your action plan flow diagram

CAN I DO ANYTHING ABOUT THIS?

YES   NO

Questions to reflect on:

1. Is this important to me and why?

2. Is this essential? Can I say no? (Dig deeper beneath 'must, should and have to'.)

3. Is this urgent? Does this really need to be done right now?

4. Is this my responsibility alone or is it shared? Can I reach out and reapportion responsibility?

5. Am I the only one who can do something about this, or can I request help/delegate?

6. What do I feel motivated or inspired to do? I can clear energetic blocks by starting here.

Based on these questions, write down now: WHAT I CAN DO, prioritizing importance, urgency and personal responsibility. Break it down into small, do-able action steps, including asking for help and nourishing your health.

Options:

Drop it like it's hot – it's ok to let this go. There is no effort, will, worry or wishing that will change this so redirect your attention to something purposeful within your control.

Acknowledge and accept this heart-breaking truth – there might be nothing of greater importance to you so you can't just drop this, but equally, you can't change it. This is when grieving begins.

Brainstorm who can help – if you can't exert influence here, who can? If you can identify someone, reach out, ask for help.

Consider ways you can make some tangible contribution – if you can't affect the outcome, what else can you do that would make a difference along the way?

Remember, it's important to take a break from problem-solving and, even if your troubles are unresolved, it's necessary to carve time to let go, drop your burden and fill up your energy bank, even if it's just for 60 seconds. We can't be productive every minute of the day and that downtime might just be the thing that helps you tap into a more creative response. Gratitude can provide a welcome relief from troubleshooting, thinking of what's gone well, or even simpler than that – what got done. If you've been in a long, drawn-out period of stress you can reflect on just how far you've come. Acknowledge all you've weathered and give yourself credit for still being on your feet. Encourage yourself just as you would a dear friend because you deserve that same tenderness. Dig deep to find those blessings in life, maybe it's the roof above your head, the profound show of love around you or the incredibly precious time that you've had. Let your mind linger there.

Choose your battles

Overcome decision-making fatigue by reducing the number of choices you have to make in your day. It can be as simple as little rituals like leaving your keys in the same place every day, having a handful of work outfits that you alternate between, choosing a time of day to exercise and sticking to it, earmarking particular evenings in the week to socialize, stocking your fridge with two different breakfasts, planning what you'll eat for lunch the next day and, even better, preparing it in advance, or rotating between five different dinners. This will free up greater willpower reserves to make difficult choices or to opt for the healthy choice, helping you beat temptation, delay gratification and tend to your future self. It's not about living a boring life with no variety, but being sensible in carving routines without reinventing the wheel daily.

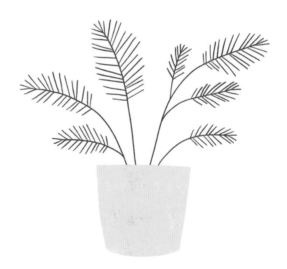

Worry time

It's normal to worry and in times of stress or crisis it would be inhumane to tell you not to worry. We do, however, need to create a container or boundary to our worries so they don't spill out and consume us. What can help is scheduling a dedicated time to worry, setting up a particular time and duration in which to fully acknowledge your concerns. While you do this, use an acupressure trick for anxiety – loosely hold your thumb in the palm of the other hand so your whole thumb is tenderly wrapped up. You can choose either hand. Be here, feeling the sensation of touch and your breath and cultivate self-compassion. Of course you feel the way you do, anyone walking in your shoes would. When your thinking is taking a downward spiral entertain the thought of other possibilities, considering not only the worst-case scenario, but the most likely and the best possible outcome too. Be proactive and jot down a couple of potential solutions to each worry. If you feel overwhelmed sifting through your worries on your own, enlist a friend who can be a safe place for you. Use your tools from the mindset section so you know how to take action that will make a difference.

When worries pop up outside of this dedicated time, remind yourself you'll have time to bear witness to them later, but it's not the time now. Worry can be persistent so we may need to draw on some powerful distraction techniques – just make sure they are life-giving ones. Opt for a walk with swinging arms to lift your mood, time in nature, use a mantra or a dip into a compelling book, or try to reframe your worries into a prayer of well wishes.

Build your pre-bedtime ritual

The mantra is 'sleep for sanity' but we all know how stress and burnout can interfere with it. Pave the way for rest and let sleep come when it will – we can't make ourselves sleep. Taking the time to drop your day before you hop into bed will help. Disentangle your mind using your mindset tools and prepare your body with this soothing sequence. Take a seat somewhere quiet, with something soft beneath you.

1. Sitting cross-legged, place your hands on your knees and make a big, fluid circling action of your torso around your hips six times before changing direction. If sitting cross-legged is uncomfortable, lie on your back, hug your knees to your chest and circle your knees around your hips instead.

2. Take a twist to rinse out the digestive system and a fold to release your hips and spine. Stretch your right leg out in front of you, flexing the right heel, bend your left knee, taking the sole of your foot inside your right knee. Breathe in and reach your arms skywards, elongating your spine. Breathe out and rotate toward your left, bringing your right hand onto your left knee and your left fingertips to the floor behind you. Stay in the twist for six breaths then, on an inhalation, come back to the centre, raising your arms up again and as you exhale, fold forward, chest toward your right knee, taking a gentle hold of your right knee or foot to anchor you. Ease yourself down into this fold without ego or strain and stay for six breaths. Slowly rise and repeat on the other side.

3. Come onto hands and knees and have a little sway. Bring your right knee toward your right hand and slide your right foot in front of your left hip. Inch your left leg back behind you, square your hips, bring your forearms to the floor and let your head surrender toward the floor. If it doesn't touch, use one or two stacked fists or your folded hands to support your forehead. Notice how nice it feels to earth your brow. Soften your legs, relax your buttocks and lengthen your exhalation. Be here for five to ten breaths before changing sides.

4. Come back to hands and knees and have one more sway, noticing the freedom and ease you've just created in your hips. Now lie down on your tummy, earthing the front of your body. Choose what feels best for you, either forehead down or turning your head to one side and supporting yourself with your hands. If you turn your head, make sure you turn it to the other side too for an equal neck release. Feel how this shape directs the breath into the back of your body. Stay for ten breaths or longer depending on your comfort. Feel free to lie on your back if you prefer. *There is nothing to be done. There is nowhere else to be.*

 Planting a seed: Have you noticed how much better you sleep after a little stretch or when you've got fresh, clean sheets? What are the things that pave the way for better sleep for you? Jot them down. What else do you notice changing in your life when your sleep is improved?

The mother of all stress busters...
one to build up to, relaxing in stillness

Having worked with the other practices to develop your mindfulness muscles and the ability to let go of your physical muscles, let's turn to the big gun...legs up the wall. There is nothing fluffy about this activity – in first aid, this is the position we bring someone into if they're in shock. It's deeply healing because it redistributes blood flow to the vital organs. I like it too as an alternative to a nap because there is no pressure to sleep and in as a little as five minutes, you've got benefit. If everyone in your care is safe, if you're comfy, it's a bonus to nod off! You might just need to set yourself an alarm.

Carve time and space to be undisturbed for the duration of this practice. Ideally you'll have 20 minutes, but even a few minutes will suffice. Set the intention to enjoy a complete absence of effort, striving or doing. Gather a blanket, an eye pillow, if you have one, and a pillow. Take a seat on the floor next to a wall, with your side facing the wall. Roll onto your back and slide your legs straight up the wall, swivelling round so the whole length of your legs is supported by it. If this creates an uncomfortable stretch in your hamstrings, sit on the floor by an armchair or sofa and take your legs up onto the seat for support instead. This diminishes the stretch but gives the same restorative effect and comfort is key. Place the pillow under your head and wrap yourself up in a blanket for comfort and warmth. Pop on your eye pillow to deepen the absence of stimulation and the gentle weight of it on your eyes is soothing.

There is nothing to achieve here. Just *flop and drop.* Allow your thoughts, feelings and memories to come and go as they will. It is not about clearing your mind but don't get absorbed in your thoughts. When inevitably you do get lost in your thoughts, don't berate yourself. Keep bringing your attention back to the physical softening of your body, the sensation of the support beneath you and your breath for a few minutes. Next, as you lie here in stillness sensing your body, extend gratitude to your body. Feel a sense of thankfulness for your organs, your brain, your heart, your skin, your hands, your legs, your spine, your calm abiding centre. It's not about appearance, it's a celebration of function over form and a deep recognition that someone else would love the body you are blessed with. Be here with your breath, feeling this sense of appreciation washing over you, cleansing you and recharging you. Stay as long as it feels good or time allows.

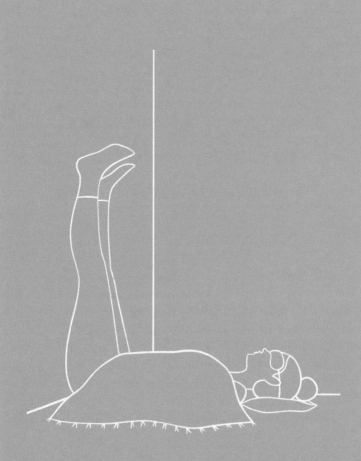

 Planting the seed: As you build the ability to relax, do you start to notice a ripple effect into your life? Are you able to respect when it is time to rest and when it's time to galvanize yourself into action? Are you better able to spot people pleasing, overachieving or other depleting behaviour? Can you extend a little more kindness your way? After time to rest, do you feel greater clarity on what matters most to you?

When I'm trying to cope/heal I will honour my energy bank basics. Have I...

- Observed my sleep needs? Or do I need to prioritize *rest for resilience* until good sleep is accessible again? In the absence of time to rest I can always *breathe better to feel better.*

- Fed and watered my mood and mental clarity?

- Moved for mental health?

- Rebooted in nature's beauty?

- Plugged in via social connection?

- Connected with my purpose? What's most important to me now?

- Checked in with myself, with tenderness?

When stressed in the moment I'll...

- Go gently on myself. Self-flagellation only adds to my burden.

- Seek ways to slow down, to close some mental tabs and reset.

- Feel the sensation of my breathing, sending it down into my belly.

- Stand tall, take a few shoulder rolls and tap into my personal power.

- Take a temporal press and reboot.

- Ask myself 'What can I do something about?' and direct my energy and attention accordingly.

- Think about something I am eagerly anticipating or imagine something pleasant, it could be as simple as my head hitting the pillow tonight!

When I'm in a crisis I'll...

- Clarify the problem, jotting down the facts of what has happened.

- Make a life map and acknowledge what's affected and what's ok.

- Notice all the emotions.

- Seek support – identify who's on my team and reach out.

- Use my existing self-care strategies to rebuild my energy and add to my toolkit if these are tricky right now.
- Minimize compensatory behaviours knowing they won't help me in the long run.
- On my own or with a partner, brainstorm potential ways to resolve the issue, identifying barriers, ways to overcome them and a simple bite-sized plan of action.

When I'm exhausted I'll...

- Acknowledge where I am at and take tender action to replenish.
- Use scent, music, colour or nature for an effortless boost.
- Draw on the power of touch to energize and sooth myself.
- Make sure I've eaten/drunk something life-giving recently.
- Schedule time for stillness or have a stretch right now.
- Plan an early night and use my pre-bedtime ritual to unwind properly.
- Use a mantra to help me through: *I soften into this moment.*

I appreciate me. This too shall pass. I give myself permission to...

When I can't sleep I'll...

- Massage some magnesium oil spray into my feet.
- Smooth out my breathing and lengthen my exhalations.
- Do some tensing and releasing of my muscles so I can access the ability to *flop and drop.*
- Soften into delicious stillness, reminding myself that it's not just sleep that's restorative – relaxation is just as good. I can also relish the knowledge that *there is nothing required of me right now.*
- Distract my mind from worry about wakefulness by remembering a happy moment.
- Scan through all the things in my life I feel grateful for.
- If sleep is elusive and I'm finding it hard to relax, I'll get up and do something soothing like floor-based stretching, listen to a guided meditation or yoga nidra. (I will not linger on any screens or stimulate my mind with worry or work – this is rest time.)

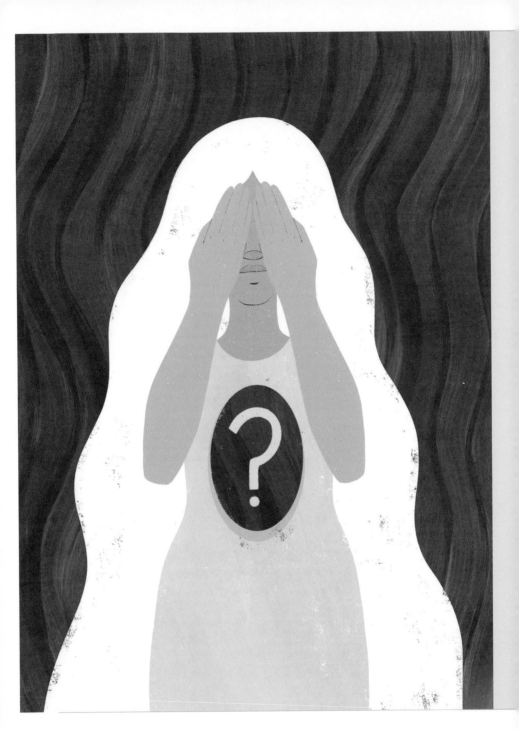

PART TWO

Loss & Grief

As we journey through life we inevitably accumulate losses, and grief is a natural part of the healing process. Broadly speaking, loss can be understood as an ending to something valued or having something or someone taken away from you and grief is the cascading of emotions in response to your loss.

WHEN DO WE FEEL LOSS & GRIEF?

Mention grief and we immediately conjure up associations of illness or death of a loved one, relationship breakdown, divorce, job loss or financial loss. There are many other life circumstances that trigger these feelings and it's important to note that these include positive and self-selected changes too, like career change, having children, retirement or moving abroad. You can grieve for a lost culture, time, place, pursuit or incarnation of you, both real and imagined. Just acknowledging the personal loss in these experiences and validating your feelings can be very healing.

Other types of loss include safety, identity, autonomy and future hopes. It may be helpful to know that for all these experiences grief is a legitimate and normal response.

» **Safety – when our emotional, mental or physical well-being has been threatened via crime or trauma, financial instability, breakdown of the family unit or betrayal, we naturally grieve our lost sense of safety.**

» **Identity – when we become parents, when our children begin school or fly the nest, when we change jobs (including promotions), voluntary positions or relationship status, when we relocate, graduate or leave home, or following a diagnosis or medical treatment like mastectomy, our feelings of identity change and we can mourn a lost role or sense of self. This is equally true whether we feel that part of our identity was taken from us or whether we embarked on a new path by choice.**

» Autonomy – we might mourn for our loss of autonomy and independence as we age, when our health is compromised, when we become parents, grandparents or carers, when we're impinged on in our careers or our financial options are limited.

» Future hopes – we grieve too for a loss of hopes and imagined futures – miscarriage, infertility, the end of a sporting career, redundancy, students struggling to carve a path once their study is complete, careers falling short of expectations, changing political climate, moving to a new country or leaving a community. Whether these are imposed or carefully chosen, you have every right to grieve what has been shed.

What do grief and loss look like and how do they feel?

Whether our loss is predicted, unexpected, sudden or prolonged, grief can be a very painful, exhausting and disorientating experience. There are many layers to it – grief can begin with the anticipation of loss, where we have time to prepare, or more suddenly when the loss is incurred without forewarning. Neither is necessarily easier and comparison seldom helps. No two losses are the same and no two healing journeys through grief are the same. Your loss is your loss and you are entitled to your feelings. There is no such thing as 'right' or 'normal' and the grieving process is deeply individual. How long it takes depends on the nature of the loss, the circumstances involved and the support available. There is no way of circumventing it or rushing through it.

All we can do is be patient with ourselves as we bear witness to our unique response to loss, reach out for support and make nourishing life choices where possible. With the passage of time, wrapped up in the love and support of people around us, things do get better, even when we feel that we or the world are forever changed.

The early stages of grief can feel like nothing you've ever experienced before. It can feel dislocating, like severe jetlag, where you feel like you're walking on a cloud, or like there's cotton wool in your head. Time might lose meaning and you may even feel like you're not in your body, watching yourself from a distance, bumbling in slow motion through this strange state of being. Grief is often characterized by waves of many different and sometimes unexpected emotions – sadness, anger, resentment, guilt, hostility and loneliness but also gratitude, love, awe and appreciation. Despite the pain, grief can pave the way for personal evolution and a renewed appreciation for life. In this ocean of feelings, the waves can be tidal in proportion at the beginning, but as time goes by, they may become smaller or less frequent, washing over us with less devastation. With the skills of mindfulness and compassion, we can learn to ride them with less overwhelm. Some people describe loss as a constant throb, an awareness that something is missing that never goes away. For others, loss feels initially deeply cutting and fades gradually with time.

You may have come across the five stages of grief proposed by Kübler-Ross[39] – denial, anger, bargaining, depression and acceptance. These might help you understand the different strands to grief but they aren't universal among the grieving, some people go through only a few of these stages and they are not in any prescribed order. The path through grief is not linear, with times of great intensity, followed by calmer times. It is normal for milestone dates and holidays to be a trigger and all those 'firsts' can be heart-breaking.

Grief potentially affects all layers of our being with a variety of mental, emotional, physical and social manifestations. It can affect our mood, outlook, memory, the ability to concentrate or think straight. We feel a raft of emotions from shock, rage, disbelief, fear and despair, to deep abiding love and thankfulness. Crying is a very normal response to loss but it's just one way of expressing yourself. Don't feel you have to cry to indicate the depth of your feeling but equally know that it's perfectly ok to show your emotion in this way. Grief can affect our energy, appetite, sleep and immune function. It can cause nausea, and aches and pains. Socially, it can affect how we feel about interacting with other people, making us want to retreat or fear being alone, and it can affect the dynamics of our relationships. It is common to feel like you're losing your mind, just plain lost, depressed, frustrated, misunderstood, ambivalent, regret for things you've done/not done/said/not said, like you want to escape, and ultimately flat as a tack. Grief can be utterly exhausting and discombobulating, and it can also feel like it is cracking you open and setting you on an unexpected path to growth, all at the same time.

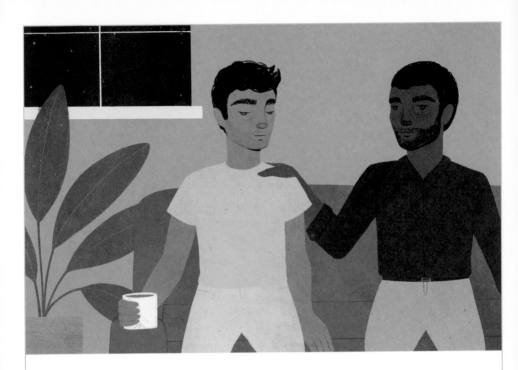

The challenge of grief is compounded by a lack of understanding about what constitutes loss and unrealistic expectations from society about how people should cope with life-changing events. Pressure to 'get over it' and a sense that we should be enjoying various chapters of life more than we do makes our grief heavier to bear. Now my children are getting older I can understand why people make the ridiculous statement 'enjoy every minute'. Any parent in the throes of those early days knows the nonsense this is. There are many experiences in life like this and we need to reclaim the right to feel the whole gamut of emotion and shake off this idea that we should swiftly move on with life after loss, or feel pressure to be happy.

Despite loss and grief being a universal experience, there is a lack of dialogue around it and real discomfort associated with the subject. People often don't know what to say or do; despite loving intentions it's easy to say the wrong thing, and often it's our fear of doing harm that leads us to say or do nothing at all. Given our deeply personal response to loss, even when you have your own lived experience, it doesn't necessarily give you insight into the kind of support someone else would like. We have to get brave and ask – ask for the help we need and ask how we can best be of support to the grieving. Some cultures have defined structure around how to navigate loss, but for many of us there are few rituals to guide us through, and we're not only learning to deal with our own emotions but also having to educate others about grief and manage their emotional response too. The notion that there are 'good' and 'bad' emotions can make grief feel more pathological, frightening and unbearable than seeing it as the normal response. And even though it is the normal response it doesn't mean that we don't need assistance in working our way through it. A greater understanding of emotional health and the tools to navigate challenging feelings will serve us all well. This is no small feat but the more we openly share with others, the more we upskill ourselves and our families, the tides will turn.

How to cope during the grieving process

- Go gently on yourself and know that it won't feel like this forever.

- Acknowledge and validate your loss.

- Give yourself permission to feel, understanding that there may be many different and unexpected emotions.

- Take the pressure off. There is no 'right' way to grieve or timeframes required.

- Reach out for support and let people know how they can genuinely help you.

- Observe your 'energy bank basics' (see page 114), use the restorative practices in the stress section to soothe your nervous system and the practices in this section to move through your emotions.

- Seek professional support if you're finding it hard to reorganize your life and reconstruct your sense of self.

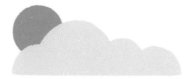

When to reach out for professional help

» If you're not sure how to handle your feelings and want support or coping strategies.

» If you don't want to be here any more.

» If you have any concerns about being depressed. It can be very hard to tell the difference between depression and grief. When you're grieving you will still experience moments of happiness and pleasure. With depression, feelings of despair and emptiness can be constant. Reach out for support from your doctor, seek out a grief counsellor or consider a support group.

» If you feel plagued by guilt or blame.

» If you're having intrusive thoughts about lost loved ones, fear about your own death or losing other people.

» If you feel numb or disconnected from others for more than a few weeks.

» If you're having trouble getting through your daily responsibilities.

WHAT ARE WE AIMING FOR?
EMOTIONAL HEALTH

To help us move through our grief it's useful to look at the building blocks of emotional health. Emotional health is the ability to understand and be responsive to our emotional experiences[40]. Being emotionally healthy is not about being happy all the time, nor are we striving to eliminate unpleasant feelings – it's the ability to feel the full range of emotions and be at ease with them. Well-being comes from being able to listen to our feelings, even the uncomfortable ones, and then attend to them responsibly. At the heart of emotional health is understanding that there's a place and purpose for all emotion and there are no positive or negative emotions – there are just emotions! Emotions act as messengers, alerting us to take action. Anger helps us take action in the face of a threat to protect ourselves or those in our care. Anxiety is there to keep us safe, alerting us to potential danger. Loneliness is a signal that we need to plug in and feel connected. Sadness is the expression of loss, signalling we need to take time out to attend to our wounds. Guilt is a reminder to check in with our moral code. We need to use our discernment and check in with the validity of these messages, and then take action accordingly – these signals might be originating from body temperature, hunger, heartbeat, muscle tension or pain and so we need to take a closer look and determine whether this is anxiety, excitement or we just need to eat something.

If we want to be emotionally healthy, we need to notice our emotions and let them move through us. That's not to say we necessarily have to take action on them, that's our choice. Emotions have an energetic charge – it's not possible to eradicate them. Think of the physical impulse you feel when you watch something funny – your body is hardwired to smile which you will feel at the corners of your lips and the crinkling of your eyes, perhaps you'll feel the eruption of a laugh. If you catch yourself and stop it, the energy doesn't just disappear. It is the same with expressions of sadness and grief. Negating, numbing or distracting ourselves from our emotions is exhausting, it creates stress, pain and tension in our bodies and disconnects us from living responsively in the moment. We can numb ourselves to our feelings but we can't do this selectively, so if we avoid the painful ones we also numb ourselves to the joyful ones too. The healthy solution is to feel what we feel and respond with mindfulness and compassion.

Emotions have an energetic charge – it's not possible to eradicate them.

Responding to our emotions in the moment

1. I'm noticing the presence of an emotion. Can I allow it to be there, getting curious about where this information might be coming from in my body? Can I sit with it rather than leaping into knee-jerk reaction? What is the message in this emotion?

2. Is this emotion appropriate to the circumstance? Is the message accurate?

3. Is this intensity appropriate to the circumstance?

4. What action might I consider taking now in response? Given my goal in this moment, is this emotion helping or hindering me? Take your time and let the emotional charge dissipate before you act.

The skills key to navigating loss and grief

Feel your emotions – to notice, allow, validate, express and move through your feelings.

Self-soothe – extending kindness and compassion toward yourself, taking tender, reparative action.

Connection – helps heal the wounds of loss and grief.

Gratitude and savouring – can transform our pain.

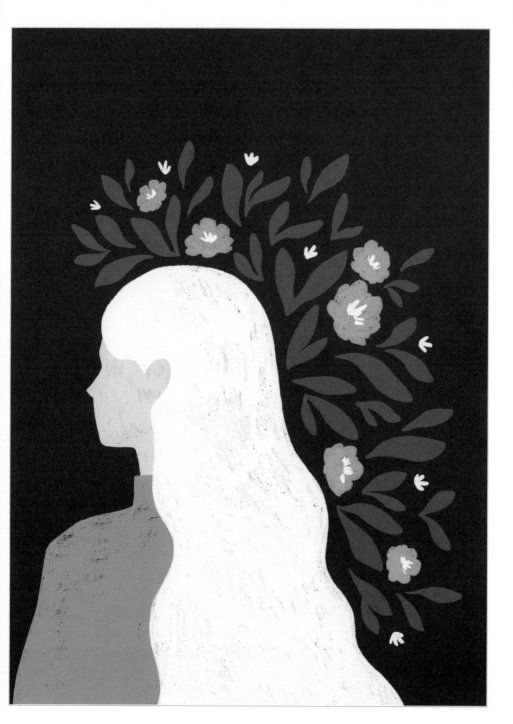

Loss & Grief

HEALING DURING TIMES OF LOSS – WHAT YOU CAN DO

SLEEP, REST, RELAXATION & BREATING – soothing practices giving me space to feel.

VALUES & PURPOSE – what do I appreciate about what's come to pass? Is this experience deepening a sense of meaning in my life?

GOALS – to allow myself to feel and be there for myself.

MOOD BOOSTERS – gratitude, savouring and welcome distractions.

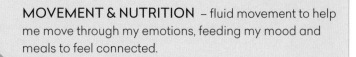

MOVEMENT & NUTRITION – fluid movement to help me move through my emotions, feeding my mood and meals to feel connected.

COPING SKILLS – developing language for emotions and the means to sit with them.

PHYSICAL ENVIRONMENT – channelling the healing power of nature and the significance of place.

SOCIAL CONNECTION – reaching out for help, building continued relationships, understanding the effects of loss on family dynamics.

THE PRACTICES FOR LOSS & GRIEF

Set the intention to go gently with these activities, being guided by your comfort and reaching out for support if you need someone to accompany you on this healing journey. The goal is to get in touch with your feelings, make space for them and to become your own safe place, while also drawing on the love and care of those around you.

Getting to know your emotions

Emotions may be a mental categorization but they originate from physical sensations in the body, so to notice and feel your emotions, you need to connect with your body. Developing this awareness will help you manage and respond to your emotions. These practices build on the body connection we developed in the stress section.

Using touch and movement to connect with your body

Another way to deepen your awareness of your body is using touch. Bodywork, like massage or acupuncture, can be powerful and with such a variety of modalities, there will be something that resonates for you. You can also engage in it yourself by simply massaging in lotion, using the massage techniques from the stress section (see page 89) or directing the flow of your shower to connect with different parts of your body.

Jaw sequence

We hold a great deal of tension in our jaw, clenching our teeth as we muscle our way through difficult experiences, or 'biting our lip' to suppress emotions. Use this sequence to let go of the things you haven't said.

1. Circle your bottom jaw around your top front teeth six times one way, then change direction.

2. Circle your bottom jaw in a round circle like you are drawing the letter 'O', six times each way.

3. This one is harder: take your bottom jaw upwards and forward and, then down and back. Then reverse it, taking your bottom jaw forward and up and then back and down. It's like an elliptical action. Do this six times each way.

4. Massage your jaw with a gentle downwards stroke a few times and notice how much more relaxed your face feels now.

 Planting a seed: Do you notice that in cultivating a physical release we also create an emotional release?

Other ways to get in touch with your emotions

Alternatives to movement and touch include watching films, reading books, reading poetry, journalling, drawing or listening to music. Try different things and see what helps you connect with your emotions.

Morning sequence – to connect, release & energize*

1. Standing check in: just notice how it feels to be standing, scanning your body and taking in what you sense. Don't worry if you don't notice much to begin with – sometimes you need to move and stretch to awaken awareness.

2. Mountain breath: stand tall with your feet hip width apart. As you breathe in, reach your arms out wide and up overhead, palms touching and looking up to lift your mood. As you exhale, bring your hands down through the centre line of your body, in prayer position, bringing the energy toward your heart. Repeat six times.

3. Shoulder rolls: fingertips on shoulders, breathe in and circle your elbows forward and upwards, exhaling to take your elbows back and down. Do six repetitions.

4. Chest and upper back release: breathe in and interlace your hands behind your back, looking up, opening your chest. Breathe out, reaching your arms forward as if you are hugging a tree and round your spine, chin to chest. Alternate between these shapes six times.

* also useful if you're feeling stuck

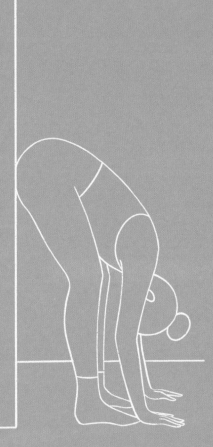

5. Standing twist: feet shoulder width apart, swing your arms and hips round to your right, looking over your right shoulder and let your left heel lift to allow a fuller twist through your spine. Swing to the left and let your right heel lift. Repeat this fluid, floppy action, letting go of any sense of effort, six times each way.

6. Forward bend against a wall: release your spine and legs with this supported forward bend. Stand with your back against the wall and your feet slightly away from the wall. Bend your knees generously and lean your lower back into the wall while you drape your spine forward along your thighs, head and hands dangling toward the floor. Flop and drop here for five to ten breaths before very slowly returning to upright.

7. Standing check in: notice now any sensations or emotional tones. Do you feel more connected with your body having moved and stretched? Does your body feel different from how it was before? You might like to pause here for a few breaths and use the mantra: '*I feel the energy circulating around my body*'.

Evening sequence – to connect, release & calm

1. Come to all fours and notice how your body feels here and now. Sway your hips from side to side several times, then turn the sway into a circle of your hips around your knees, six times one way, feeling this oil the hip joint, then change direction.

2. Wide Child's pose: take your knees wide apart, big toes touching, sink your bottom to your heels, chest, forearms and forehead toward the floor. Let your forehead rest on the floor or fold your hands or make a fist to provide support. Soften and drop, feeling how it is to be in this shape.

3. Swimming Child's pose: from the shape above, as you breathe in, sweep your right arm back behind you and rise to all fours with your right arm arcing up and over like front crawl. Exhale back to Wide Child's pose. As you breathe in, take your left arm back behind you and rise again to all fours with the left arm swimming up and over. Repeat six times each side, allowing your chest to turn with the movement and watching your hand with your gaze. Feel this open the side body and immerse yourself in the sensation of moving in time with your breath.

4. Down Dog: from all fours, tuck your toes under, raise your hips up and press your heels back and down, coming into an upside-down 'V' shape. Your legs needn't be straight, the priority is a long spine. Hold for five to ten breaths, connecting with the sensations of this pose. Return to Wide Child's pose to rest and refresh.

5. Thread the Needle: from a Wide-knee Child's pose, lift up to all fours. Breathe in, raise your right arm skywards and look up. Exhale and thread your right arm underneath your left, along the floor, taking your right ear to the floor. Repeat six times before changing sides.

6. Rest in a shape of your choosing – Child's pose, on your tummy, on your back, and observe how you feel now, any sensation or emotion. Use the mantra: '*the energy of the universe supports and protects me*'.

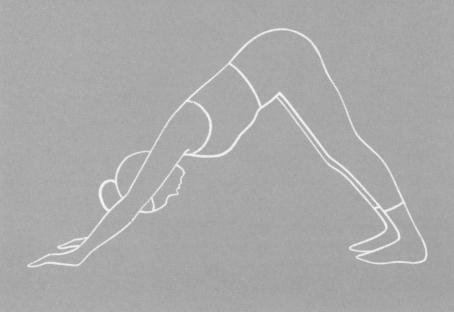

Loss & Grief

UNDERSTANDING YOUR EMOTIONS

The first step to understanding your emotions is having rich vocabulary to describe them. Language creates a link between experience and thought so to be able to make sense of your emotions you need the words to describe and categorize them. The vocabulary we have to label emotion helps us develop 'emotional literacy'[41] – being able to label our emotion accurately, and the breadth of experience of different emotions is called 'emotional granularity'[42] – rather than just feeling 'bad', being able to describe the shades of different feelings like boredom, frustration or disappointment, helps us take more targeted action and move through it. Research shows that possessing broad language and the ability to finely distinguish between difficult feelings makes it easier to regulate your emotions, to respond more constructively and with greater flexibility[43]. These skills are good for our health – people who have higher emotional granularity are less likely to drink excessively when stressed[44] and can be less prone to retaliate with aggression when provoked[45]. Being skilled at differentiating between emotions also allows us to reframe how we feel with greater effect, so, for example, reframing nervousness as anticipation.

Take in this list of different emotions. Look up the definition of any you are unsure of. What might their purpose be? Are there some that you try to avoid? Why might this be? How would it be if you made space for these emotions?

Love   Courage   Vigilance   Remorse

Admiration   Power   Annoyance   Gloom

Awe   Zest   Irritation   Unease

Joy   Playfulness   Alarm   Mortification

Bliss   Gratitude   Anger   Rejection

Elation   Contentment   Rage   Embarrassment

Inspiration   Happiness   Shock   Resentment

Openness   Relaxation   Fear   Envy

Hope   Serenity   Worry   Jealousy

Eagerness   Pride   Anxiety   Disappointment

Amazement   Excitement   Disgust   Loneliness

Astonishment   Anticipation   Boredom   Guilt

Acceptance   Interest   Apathy   Dismay

Amusement   Curiosity   Sadness   Tetchiness

Peace   Nervousness   Melancholy

 Planting a seed: Does a broader vocabulary help you understand your emotions better and acknowledge what you need in different moments? Does it allow you to express yourself more confidently?

Making peace with your emotions

Your inner commentary about your emotions can help you relax into your experience or can amplify your discomfort. This physical sequence will develop your understanding of how judgement shapes your subjective experience.

1. First warm up your body either by taking a walk around the block or use the evening sequence from this section (see page 136).

2. Locate a small towel and lie down on the floor with something soft beneath you. Hug your knees into your chest and have a little rock from side to side.

3. Stretch your legs out long and come into an awareness of your body. Without judgement of whether it is 'good' or 'bad', just notice how you feel lying in stillness.

4. Keeping your left leg long and heel flexed to engage it like an anchor, hug your right knee into your chest, hook the tea towel around the ball of your right foot and stretch your right foot skywards. You will notice a stretch in the back of your right leg which

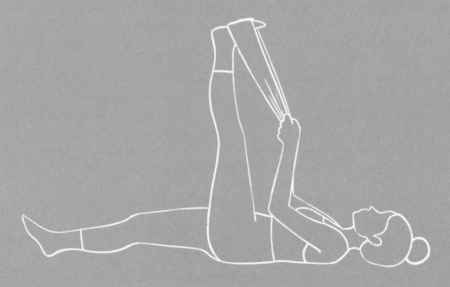

deepens the straighter you have your leg. You are in control of this intensity. Work your legs as straight as you can, making sure that you can breathe comfortably. Focus all your attention on the sensation in the back of your right leg, noticing what happens when you make your breathing slower and more spacious. As you relax into your breathing, does this take some of the edge off the sensation or make it somehow more bearable? Notice with time how the sensation changes and maybe you can straighten the leg even further? Don't overstretch, it is essential that we can breathe smoothly and there are no benefits in pushing past your comfort zone. Hold here for ten slow breaths, noticing your tendency to want to label your experience. Critical thoughts about your ability or judgements about the experience itself, like 'this is painful/awful, I want it to stop', all tend to amplify discomfort. Softening your dialogue, tapping into curiosity – 'I wonder what would happen if I...' – or reframing this from 'unpleasant' to 'significant' or 'intense' helps you make peace with the sensation. Judgement makes us recoil, fighting the experience, keeping us stuck, whereas openness helps us soften into it and accept it, allowing it to move through us. What we are developing here is self-compassion and the ability to self-soothe.

5. Release the stretch and notice that the sensation doesn't go on forever – it had a beginning and an end and we had some control over it by using relaxed breathing and choosing our inner dialogue wisely. Repeat the stretch on your left leg, immersing yourself in the sensations and the impact your thoughts and words have on how it feels. Notice how you feel afterwards too – the release for your legs and spine. It may have been intense but the release can feel pleasant.

6. We can work with our emotions in the same way. Just like sensations, our emotions are transient and we can shape our experience of them. Know it will pass. Allow them to arise, experience them openly and watch them fade. Get curious, relax into your breath, speak to yourself with tenderness – it is still intense but there's less struggle. Try using the mantra: *'I make peace with my feelings'*.

 Planting a seed: As I build this tolerance for physical sensation, can I approach emotional anguish in the same way? This may take considerable practice so go gently and start small. To further empower you, build some toolkits to manage your emotions, like those at the end of this section. When I am feeling 'X', I will...

Boosting your digestion

This practice supports physical digestion and can help us release our emotions too. Warm your hands by rubbing them together then place your fingertips by your right hip, press them up towards the ribcage, across your abdomen and down towards your left hipbone, across your lower abdomen and back to your right hip. Repeat the circling action in this direction for a few minutes while lengthening your exhalation, maybe through pursed lips, like you're blowing out a candle. You may hear and feel gurgles in your tummy. Next hug your right knee into your chest, pressing it firmly against your tummy, and let it go. Alternate legs, repeating this ten times. This is affectionately known in yoga as the 'wind-relieving' pose, so don't be surprised if you hear more rumbles. Relax your legs into a position comfortable for you, place one hand on your heart, one on your belly, feeling your breath, the warmth of your hands and extend towards yourself a feeling of care. Use the mantra '*I am my own safe place*'.

Lion breath

Sometimes we need to expunge ourselves of big emotions like anger, resentment and frustration. The challenge is to do this in ways that are not harmful. Roaring it out in lion breath can help, akin to screaming into a pillow. Breath in through your nose, exhale with an explosive 'ha' sound through your mouth, sticking your tongue out as far as possible, three times. Blow away what is hard or harmful to say.

Practices to soothe – book openings

Lying on your back, with a pillow beneath your head, on the floor or in your bed, just feel your breathing for a minute. Don't worry if it feels short or tight and don't work to make it any different than you find it. Next, turn onto your left-hand side with your arms out at chest height and your knees bent, roughly in line with your hips. Imagine your body is like a closed book in this position. As you breathe in, peel your right arm slowly back behind you and follow it with your gaze. As you breathe out, return to your starting position, closing the pages of the book. Repeat this six times, noticing that with each repetition your chest muscles loosen a little more and maybe your arm drops back a little further. Repeat this on the other side and then return to your back, feeling the expansiveness of your breath across your chest and how comforting this feels. Is your breath a little slower now too? Notice how calming it is when your rate of breathing slows down.

 Planting a seed: When we are trying to avoid emotions or hold them down, our breath tends to become very small and our body becomes tight. Notice how freeing it feels to move with the breath, and to let the breath feel bigger and more spacious. In time, perhaps this might help you make space for your emotions and move through them, taking them literally one breath at a time.

Practices to soothe – meditation on your heart centre

Come into a comfortable position with your spine elongated, on a chair or a meditation cushion. Close your eyes, soften the muscles of your face and shoulders and take a few relaxed breaths. As you breathe in, take your fingertips to touch behind the base of your skull, exhale and slowly move them forward around your head, without touching your head, meeting at the centre of your forehead, palms touching. Breathe in here and then slowly move your hands to your heart, keeping the palms together in prayer shape. As you repeat this action of your hands, imbue it with the intention to gather your mental energy at the centre of your forehead and bring it down into your heart. You may even begin to feel a sense of energy or warmth between your hands as you press them together and a sense of this energy moving into your heart centre. After a few minutes pause with your hands one on top of the other across your heart. Breathe into them and imagine in your heart centre a ball of white light, a candle burning or the sun rising over the ocean. Let your mind's eye linger on this image of light and feeling of warmth emanating from your heart. Breathe in more light and life and exhale away what you no longer need. Use the mantra: '*I can be there for myself*'.

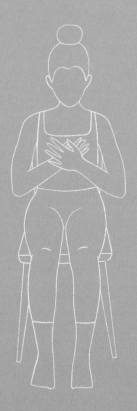

 Planting a seed: Whenever your thoughts are scattered or your energy feels dissipated, use this practice to centre yourself and re-enter your day anchored in purpose.

The importance of connection

'What we once enjoyed and deeply loved we can never lose. For all that we love deeply becomes a part of us.'[46]
– Helen Keller

When I lost my father to motor neurone disease, second only to the pain of seeing him suffer, was the pain of lost connection. It's not only death that can leave us feeling disconnected, but physical distance, conflict, ruptures in relationships or just feeling out of kilter can all leave us feeling raw.

Connection is the balm that soothes the pain of grief – feeling the loving face to face care of your tribe around you and building a sense of continued relationship with what or who you have lost. On a simple level, when I hung up my figure skates after a childhood of dedication, turning to yoga gave me a similar sense of expression in a form I could sustain for the rest of my days. I also relished working as a psychologist with young skaters. My love for the sport and presence in the community could evolve and this soothed my sense of loss.

On a more profound level, creating a continued relationship with my father helped me cope and heal following his passing. Thinking that my father is gone forever is something I still can't get my head around. The pain of that separation feels unbearable but what I have come to appreciate is that this is a self-imposed notion of distance. We don't have to be torn asunder. Yes, he is no longer here in earthly form, but I am made from the cells and fibres of his body and my mother's body, so we can never truly be apart. We are one and the same. I think this is true for any being you've come to love, family or not. We become delicately interwoven and that connection transcends space and time. By thinking about my father, remembering silly moments, happy anecdotes, little flashbulb memories, I can conjure his loving presence and feel wrapped up in it. I can stay current with him by talking about him with my kids, sharing moments with him in a little prayer, going out for a run as he loved to do, or heading out into nature's beauty as we so often did together. He is still very much here with me and our connection lives on.

How can we create continued relationships?

Ask for reminiscences from family and friends – it could be a couple of lines, a story that illuminates who they were or what they stood for or a photograph. Collate these tributes into a book of memories, forming a celebration of their life and legacy, and a touchstone to feel their continued presence.

Engage in activities you loved doing together – it could be preparing a meal you enjoyed, allowing the power of scent and taste to transport you. Share these recipes with your family to keep that lineage alive.

Write a letter – express anything left unsaid, say it out loud or send a prayer.

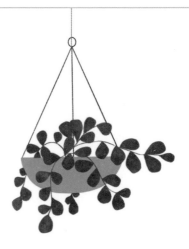

Is there a place that helps you feel close? Perhaps it's an environment that reminds you of them, somewhere you enjoyed visiting together, a familiar coffee shop, a bench or the location of a specific memory. Perhaps your loved one leaves calling cards, like a feather, or visits you in different forms, like a bird or a butterfly. I've been stopped in my tracks by a kingfisher three times since Dad died – the day of his funeral, the day my son started nursery and a day when I had an intense grief counselling session. His message was unmistakeable. When that deep longing arises, visit these significant places and remember times spent there. What would you say to them now? Feel embraced by their loving energy. Even if you can't physically visit these places you can use photographs or go there in your mind and visualize the same experience.

 Planting a seed: Your relationship continues and it is anchored in your body and in the landscape around you – touch in with it whenever you can. Does this diminish the feeling of separation or space between you?

The effects of death on family dynamics

While talking about connection it is important to touch on how bereavement can affect those left behind. We need to remember that grief affects us all differently, so do your best to avoid judgement or comparison. Grief can make us all feel raw, sensitive and vulnerable and when we are hurting we are sometimes less able to censor ourselves, speaking and behaving in ways that we wouldn't ordinarily. The mantra 'hurt people hurt people' might be useful to remember in navigating bereavement and your relationships with others who are bereaved. The aftermath of death can be a pressure cooker situation with delicate arrangements to be made and estates to settle, often the seeds for conflict. Things can feel very different in a family or group when someone is not physically there any more, dynamics might change, people might change and relationships might change. Compassion all round is key.

 Planting a seed: Sometimes the relationships that normally sustain us are compromised in the wake of loss. Seek support from a variety of sources, from within the family unit and from your broader circle. Let people know how they can help and give yourself permission to shape the nature of your social interactions. The loving presence of animals which I affectionately term 'pet therapy' can also be deeply soothing at these times.

LIFTING YOUR SPIRITS

The burden of grief can be overwhelming so we need to both face our feelings of loss and know when and how to take a break and find an oasis of calm between the storms of grief. These can also help you dig beneath your sadness, revealing the presence of many other emotions that in time can transform your pain.

Welcome distractions and mood-boosting skills

Give yourself permission to take a break from grief – anchor your mind on anything you find nourishing – making or listening to music, creating or appreciating art, scrapbooking, knitting, Sudoku, card games, board games, your favourite comedy, walking the dog, meditating on nature, movement, tidying, touch, scent, time with friends, volunteering, your resource library (see page 74), mantra or your breath.

Savouring – this is the ability to drink in joyful experiences and it's a powerful mood booster, because comingled with your feelings of loss are also feelings like thankfulness, appreciation and love. Savouring will help you notice and reap the benefits of lighter and breezier feelings. You can savour the past by sifting through happy memories, reliving them in your mind's eye, in a letter or in conversation. You can savour the present by bearing witness to current blessings, using

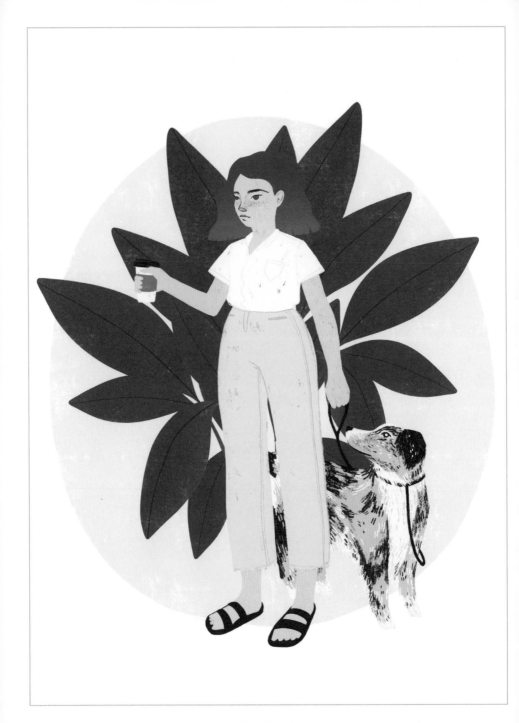

Loss & Grief

all of your senses. It can be as simple as the ritual of tea in a teacup you love. You can savour the future by using the power of your imagination to anticipate possible experiences of contentment and peace, reminding yourself that life won't always feel this heavy and hope is a powerful motivator to keep going.

Gratitude, appreciation, awe and admiration – beneath your feelings of loss you will have a great reservoir of thanks and love to mine. Allow your mind to linger on what it is that you loved so much about what's come to pass – the moments, the memories, the lessons, the qualities. In time to come, you may find that your pain is transformed into these emotions, allowing you to wholeheartedly embrace life in its new shape.

Purpose and meaning – while initially loss can feel confusing, with the passage of time it also has the potential to connect you deeply with what matters most in life, refining how and where you spend your energy. Reflecting on how this experience is encouraging you to grow and the insights gleaned into your strengths and values can help you move forward in your healing journey.

 Planting a seed: When you are feeling overwhelmed by loss, allow yourself an uplifting break. This is an important part of reconstructing your own sense of self. Remember that underneath your grief is enormous love – let that flood through you too.

TOOLKITS

When I am in pain I'll...

- Bear witness, allowing myself to feel as I do.

- Befriend my pain – this is what healing feels like.

- Ask myself how any other human being would feel in my shoes and extend tenderness toward myself as I would a loved one.

- Cry, howl, roar it out with lion breath, move with it, or be quiet and still.

- Notice the texture and sensation, tuning into my physical body, softening into it, listening to the wisdom of body.

- Repeat the mantra *I am safe, I am loved, I am held*. The earth holds me. I can turn to others for love and comfort. I hold myself. I am here for myself.

- Remember: I am worthy. I am entirely lovable as I am now. What I bring to this world is valuable.

- Turn to my Vitality Wheel for self-soothing inspiration, taking one step at a time on my healing journey, at my own pace.

- Reach out for help and I can shape how that support is given.

- Take solace in the knowledge that this feeling will pass. From this pain, insight and evolution can come.

When I'm tearful I'll...

- Remember my loss is real.

- Give myself permission to acknowledge and mourn it.

- Allow my tears to fall now if this is an appropriate time. If not, I will respect my feelings but carve out space to express them more fully later. I can draw on touch, mantra and my breath right now to help me move through this and carry on with my day.

When I'm missing someone I'll...

- Honour this as a desire to feel connected and to express my love.

- Give thanks for the blessing this person was and still is to me, thinking about what they taught me or how they helped me become who I am today.

- Look for ways to plug in and experience a sense of loving presence whether that's using a photograph, memories or drawing on nature and place.

- Think about other people in my life who can fill this need right now and reach out.

- Remind myself that I can provide comfort and safety for myself too.

When I feel sad about the end of a chapter I'll...

- Allow myself to feel sad, knowing I can't hide from my feelings or outrun them.

- Remember that every moment I am hurting, I am doing the work of healing. The only way out is through.

- Reframe my view of sadness or pain, knowing it's not out to get me

or take over my life, it has meaning and purpose. It is a testament to my love for what has come to pass and I honour it. What is it telling me I need today?

When I feel anger or resentment for what I've been through I'll...

- Acknowledge my right to feel it – this is how I stand up for myself and my values, maintain my boundaries and keep myself safe.

- Express it in a constructive way, using movement, breathing, powerful venting on a piece of paper that I will relish throwing away, or out loud (out of earshot) with some cathartic swearing.

- Create some boundary to it so it doesn't keep burning away, which only harms me in the long run. I'll feel it and let it go, using welcome distractions if I need to.

- Spend some time reflecting on the concept of forgiveness – myself, others and life itself, knowing we forgive to free ourselves, not for the transgressor and it does not condone the wrongdoing.

- Return to my energy bank basics to replenish myself (see page 114).

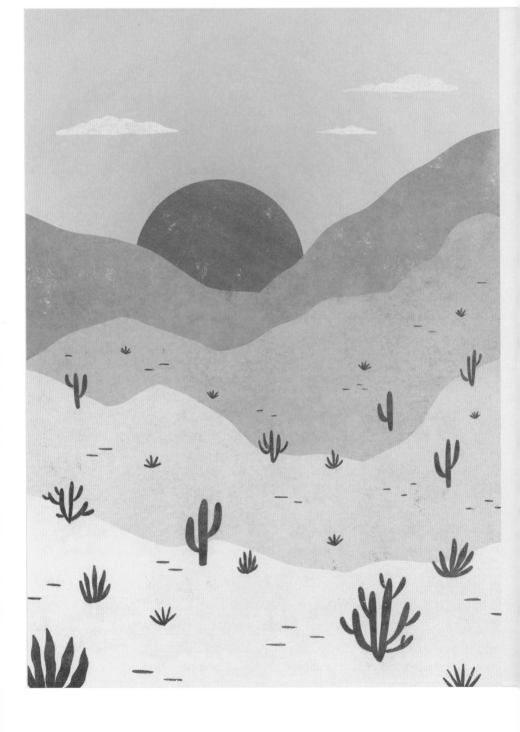

PART THREE

Change & Transition

Change is happening within us and all around us. Every day we wake with a different mind and body thanks to neural plasticity and cellular renewal, immersed in a different environment with seasonal ebb and flow. Despite it being the one constant in life, the dynamics and implications of change and transition are poorly understood. Like grief, we just don't talk about it enough, but this is slowly changing. The word 'matrescence' was first used in the 1970s to describe the transition into motherhood but it's only in the last few years that this concept has entered the public domain, recognizing the challenges unique to this time of life[47]. There is nothing new about menopause, but again it is only recently becoming less of a taboo subject. Retirement is another major life transition that is commonly misunderstood, with a spate of recent research[48] showing that we're finally getting this on the radar too.

CHANGE & TRANSITION – HOW ARE THEY DIFFERENT?

Change and transition are terms often used interchangeably and this is one of the reasons why navigating them can be so difficult. William Bridges[49] makes an insightful and useful distinction between the two:

» **Change refers to the situation or external factors.**

» **Transition refers to the psychological factors, the inner reorientation, redefining of self and reorganization of life in response to change.**

For a transition to be successful we have to make the necessary inner shifts, which may involve a shedding, a loss of some kind to be acknowledged and mourned. According to Bridges there are three components of transition:

» **An ending – we need to let go of the old before we can move on. This can be like an experience of dying – the end of us or life as we know it. Recognizing this ending and allowing ourselves to grieve is fundamental to navigating change and transition. I hope you find this as freeing as I did. It makes sense that we mourn this loss of identity, letting go of a belief, attitude, habit, activity (like breastfeeding), chapter, relationship (even when the relationship is intact but the dynamic changes, such as when your child is no longer a baby), role, vision or dream.**

» The neutral zone – the chapter between the old and the new, a period often characterized by confusion, distress, shapelessness and emptiness.

» A new beginning – a new sense of self is born, new rhythms and patterns of life are emerging, refreshed purpose, direction and action, a feeling of resonance and coming home to yourself.

Why it's challenging

It doesn't matter if it's positive change, change of your choosing or change that's out of your control – it's still challenging. It is made more difficult with modern society's preoccupation with change and scant reference to transition. There's no road map, there are few societal milestones or rites of passage. We all find this inner reorientation hard and it's normal to feel like a part of us is fighting to defend our old self as if our life depends on it. We tend to rush through transition, technology fuelling in us a desire for instant gratification, we're becoming more impatient and unable to wait. There's a fundamental disrespect for fallow time and inactivity is seen as laziness. FOMO and the 'you snooze you lose' mentality drive us to leap before we're truly ready, propelling us into action for the illusion of productivity. It is true, incompletions are draining and unfinished business depletes us, but we can't rush or force our way through the inner shift required to make it successfully through to a 'new normal'.

What it can feel like

There's often stress, loss and grief in the process of change and transition. It can be devastating and painful, confusing and seemingly nonsensical. When we recognize there's an ending, of course we grieve, for the loss of our own childhood, for our capacities, autonomy and independence, as we move through the seasons of our life, as we watch our children grow and journey to independence, as we embark on new careers, relationships, pursuits or uproot ourselves.

Among the feelings of fear, discomfort and sadness there is also exhilaration, excitement, liberation and the celebration of rebirth! Variety is the spice of life, and change is fertile ground for growth. Transition is the very stuff personal evolution is made of.

Change and transition feel very much like cycles: a time of letting go, liminal space like a gestation period, then stepping up and a feeling of becoming or coming into your own, followed by another letting go. You might also feel like it's an alternation between expansion and contraction, a process of disintegration and reconstruction, or death and rebirth.

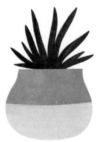

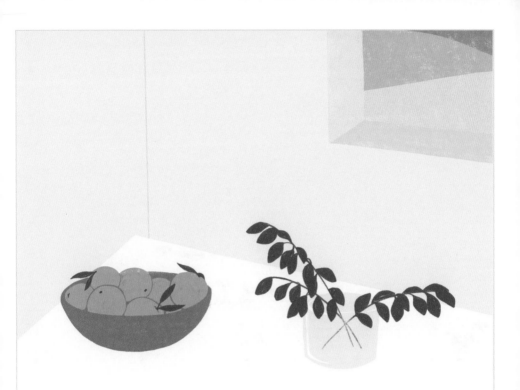

The skills key to navigating change and transition

Patience and tolerance for ambiguity – the ability to sit with the discomfort of change, the loss, the shapelessness, the not knowing, the parts that are beyond your control and the process that can't be expedited.

Self-insight – knowing yourself, that part of you that remains unchanged, identifying your strengths and values.

Courage and strength – the bravery to have your own back and advocate for yourself, facilitating targeted and purposeful action.

COPING WITH CHANGE & TRANSITION – WHAT YOU CAN DO

SLEEP, REST, RELAXATION & BREATHING – long exhalations to help navigate an ending, alternate nostril breathing for balance in the neutral zone, ujjayi breathing (see page 165) for resolve during a new beginning.

VALUES & PURPOSE – making sense of change, post-traumatic growth, creating a life aligned with what matters most to you, being of service.

GOALS – get to know your future best self, understanding goals and willpower, reflecting on your accomplishments, praising effort not just outcome, recognizing how far you've come and what you've weathered.

MOOD BOOSTERS – curiosity, playfulness, laughter.

MOVEMENT & NUTRITION – seasonal eating, playing with novelty, using posture for confidence.

COPING SKILLS – acceptance and 'right effort', thinking constructively about change and your developing identity.

PHYSICAL ENVIRONMENT - nature as the guru of change.

SOCIAL CONNECTION – new connections, reaching out to people who inspire you and mentoring.

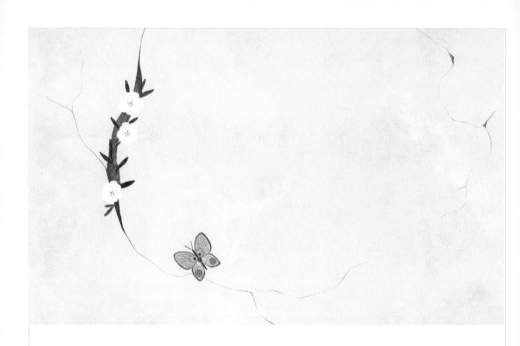

THE PRACTICES FOR CHANGE & TRANSITION

Integral to the process of navigating change and transition is the ability to relax and soothe your mind and body which we explored in the section on stress, and the ability to acknowledge your loss and to feel and move through your emotions which we explored in the section on grief. You may find it useful to develop those skills first before diving into the practices in this section, but if you feel energized, resolved and motivated you can start right here. Building on the practices from the sections on stress and grief, we have new ones to explore – to help us accept change and transition, to develop greater insight into ourselves as we forge a new identity and to help us carve a path of purposeful action.

Making peace

Just as we made space for our sensations and emotions, we now turn our attention to softening into our experience of change and transition. Play with these different ways of becoming more comfortable with change and transition:

Nature as the guru of change

If you want to understand and appreciate the full spectrum of change in all its glory, turn to Mother Nature. She has so many metaphors that we can draw on to make sense of and make peace with life's unfolding events. Take one look at the tenacity of nature to survive and even thrive in the most harrowing of conditions and you're reminded of the same strength of the human spirit. Reflect on the flower that blooms from the tiny crack in the pavement, making use of every resource available; we can be just as capable and grateful. The willow that bends and sways with the turbulence of the wind; we can be just as resilient and malleable. The eruption of new life following a forest fire; in the aftermath we can blossom similarly. Just as the butterfly bides its time, emerging from the chrysalis when ready, not a moment too soon, we can give ourselves the gift of time. The farmer knows to rest his field, deeply respecting the need for fallow time. The seasons remind us of the impermanence of life, that there is a time for all things and there is beauty and purpose in all stages – the promise of the bud, the attractiveness and pollination of the bloom and the decaying petals, returning to the earth to nourish the next flower.

Reflecting on nature we can see that this is just the way things are, and there is no changing it. We have no choice but to cultivate acceptance because no effort, will or wishing will make a difference and fighting it only leads to your depletion[50]. Draw on nature's messages to help you soften into that knowing, allowing it is to be as it is. It can be uncomfortable, it can be painful and it can be liberating in time too. Meditate on nature and learn to sit with it. Try this ritual to connect with the seasons of life – cut some flowers from the garden, appreciating their origin. Relish their beauty and imbibe the sustenance they offer in this phase. As the petals fall, use them to make a mandala, appreciating them in this form. Then toss them back to enrich the earth. Growing a vegetable or herb garden can embed us in this same natural process. Some mantras to support you: '*I give myself time. There is time!*', '*I honour the fallow period. Nothing blooms all year*', '*I savour the joyful and make peace with the painful*'.

What we eat

On a simple level, we can get into the rhythm of change by observing seasonal flow, choosing foods sourced locally. We can become more accustomed to change by trying new foods and beverages, making different meals or new recipes, and sampling foods from different cultures.

Using the breath

We can use the breath in different ways to support us through each phase of a transition.

Making your exhalations long – try this to help you let go and move through an ending.

Alternate nostril breathing – can be calming and balancing,[51] anchoring us while we are in the neutral zone.

This can also be useful for tension headaches. Place the first two fingers of your dominant hand between your eyebrows. You'll use the pad of your thumb and the inner tip of your ring finger to alternately close one nostril. Begin by closing your right nostril and breathing in through your left nostril. Close your left nostril and breathe out through your right. Breathe in through your right, then breathe out through your left. Breathe in through your left and out through your right again, changing nostrils after each breath in. Repeat this for up to five minutes and always complete the practice by exhaling through your left nostril. If sleep is elusive you can try alternate nostril breathing or even imagining it can help soothe your nervous system.

Ujjayi breathing – can support you as you embark on a new beginning because it is both energizing and comforting[52]. In ujjayi breathing, you breathe in and out through the nose with the back of the throat partially closed, as if you are saying with word 'ha' but with closed lips, and the inhalation and exhalation are of equal length. You'll hear a subtle sound like the ocean or perhaps akin to Darth Vader, feeling the breath delicately stroke the back of your throat, without any tension in your tongue, jaw, throat or neck. Aim for a few minutes and turn to this practice wherever and whenever you like, avoiding it when you are congested.

Observing how we think

Observe any tendency toward comparison – both between yourself and others and between your 'old' and 'current' self. Notice how it affects you. This is just a habit and you can learn to drop it if doesn't serve you.

Climb out of the vortex of 'why' and step into the power of 'what' – in times of change we can get lost in a sea of whys. Notice when your mind is drawn to these endless questions and bring it back to something more constructive, focusing on what you can do.

Be careful with the words you choose – they have great power. Reframe 'I have to' to 'I get to' or 'I choose to'. Switch 'I can't' for 'I don't'.

Remember that it won't be like this forever – even when there is no end in sight. You may find some solace in the words 'this too shall pass'.

 Planting a seed: What's your relationship with change and transition? Is it new to you that there is a distinction between them? Do these definitions help you understand why it's been so tough? Separating them out, how do you feel about the outer trappings of change – the external variables, and what comes to mind when you think about the stages of transition – the ending, the limbo state, the new beginning? You might have a different relationship with each. Plot a timeline of all the significant changes in your life and reflect on how these experiences have shaped your relationship with change and transition. If you find yourself thinking negatively, from your own experiences, how can you broaden this thinking?

GETTING TO KNOW YOURSELF: PAVING THE WAY FOR REBIRTH

What does identity mean to you?

Who are you in the midst of all this change? Our identity is often tied up with names, appearance, skills, interests, pastimes, gender, sexuality, education, career, relationship status, financial standing, community, nationality, ethnicity, religion, language, culture and political persuasion. But what lies underneath? What are the constants? What is your true nature, that which remains the same regardless of outer variables? The beauty of sitting in the 'no man's land' of transition is that these things can become clearer. In all the activities where we watched our sensations, emotions and thoughts, observing their transience, did you start to connect with the constant part of you? The part that witnesses, the part that is unsullied by any event? You can think of it as your divine self or maybe consciousness itself. You are more than your story. You are more than the hats you wear. What lies beneath all the roles and responsibilities you own? We are shaped by our life events but we don't need to be defined by them.

Take some time to think about how you define yourself and reflect on the interconnectedness of life. Find a bench to sit on and watch the hum of life around you. Observe with all your senses, the aromas, the sounds, the sights, the tastes, the textures and the memories these evoke. Let it all wash over you, noticing the movement of people around you – people like you, sitting and watching the world go by, acknowledging your shared experience. Notice people walking, running, driving, on buses, trains or planes. Reflect on the times you've taken those modes of transport and the places you've been, connecting with that feeling of common purpose. Notice the goings on around you, without judgement, and think about when have you've had similar experiences. Feel that deep sense of shared humanity and let your mind linger on the notion that you, like every human being, are an integral part of this whole picture. See how it feels to rely less on things outside of you to define you. Feel this natural sense of connectedness with the world, belonging to something bigger than yourself, your place in it, everyone's place in it. You matter. Everyone matters. Alternatively, you could contemplate the cosmos and see how this is reflected in the intricacies of the human body, even the structure of a cell, or you could just gaze at the stars.

Write a letter to you, choosing the prompts that resonate for you. What do you want to say to yourself? What do you need to hear?

Plot a timeline of your life events – review your achievements and include what you have weathered. How would anyone walking in your shoes feel?

Look to the positive – what qualities do you appreciate about yourself?

Reflect on your current situation – what are you currently doing well? Praise not only positive outcomes but effort, tenacity, grit, showing up, persistence or care.

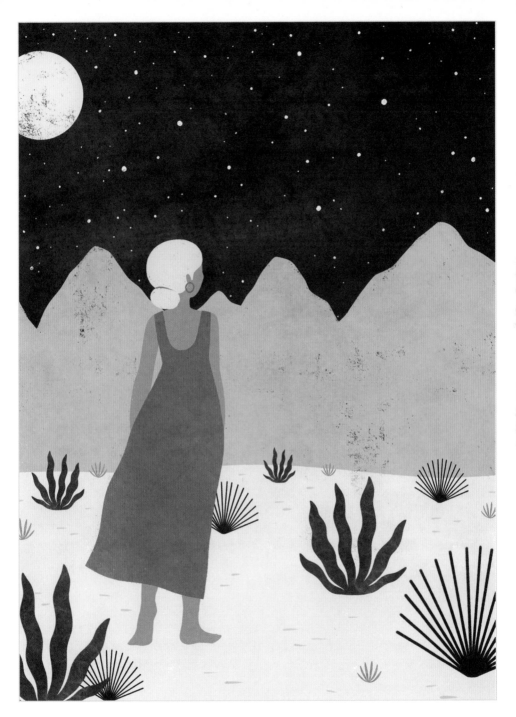

Change & Transition

Explore your fears – acknowledge why they are concerns for you. When do you feel at ease and why? Our ability to relax is more than just our muscle fibres, it is also found in congruence, that feeling of peace when we are aligned with our values. Use this information to reflect on what you feel your purpose is.

Make a commitment – ensure you honour what's important to you, including looking after to you. What might that look like?

IDENTIFY YOUR STRENGTHS & VALUES

Your strengths are things you do well naturally and effortlessly and your values are what matters most in life to you. They both light us up and motivate us. We feel powerful when we put our strengths to good use and we can call on them to help us navigate tough times. Knowing our values helps us connect with a sense of meaning in challenging times.

Play with the following methods to gain greater self-insight:

- Who do you feel a resonance or connection with? Why?

- Who do you admire (these can be people in your life, celebrities, historical figures or fictional characters)? Why?

- What are your proudest moments, and why? What qualities did you draw on?

- If money was no issue, how would you spend your time?

- If you had nothing to fear what action would you take or what would you stop doing?

- Reflect on what makes you angry, what underlying morals are being impinged on?

- Search online for 'Values in Action' and take the 'Character Strengths Survey' which will rank for you 24 strengths. The top five are what you do well, the bottom five are potential points for improvement if you choose.

- Journal about the different roles you play in life and look at the deeper qualities you aspire to possess in those roles. How do you want to be experienced? What would you like to model for others? How would you like to be remembered?

Post-traumatic growth[53] and meaning

One of the ways we can make sense of change and pave the way for the emergence of our new sense of self is to dig beneath our pain to see the ways that we are growing as a result of this challenge. The following questions might help you find some meaning in the chaos, and once the dust has settled might reveal a silver lining to your struggle:

- How is this experience developing your perception of who you are, your capabilities, your purpose?

- What lessons are you learning about life or the world?

- Have new doors opened as a result of this challenge?

- Are there relationships that are deepening as a result?

- Is this experience cultivating a feeling of appreciation for precious aspects of your life, for life itself?

 Planting a seed: In tough times, ask yourself, what are you learning about yourself, about others, about the world? Can you reframe this as an opportunity to grow, to develop a quality that you hold dear? Zoom out and see if you can perceive a bigger picture, this circumstance anchored in greater perspective. Can you also extend toward yourself a huge dollop of tenderness and compassion – this is tough and it hurts, any human being would find it so.

CARVING YOUR PATH OF ACTION

We've talked at length about surrender, acceptance and making peace but there is time for action too. You are not just a passive recipient of life. You can be powerful, creative and resourceful in response to life and you choose where you place your energy, attention and effort. The key is identifying where your control lies, what's genuinely important to you and your available resources. Create your life map (see page 104) to get started and use the following exercises to bring focus and clarity to your next steps.

Mindful ritual

Come into a seated position and ease out any tension in your neck, chest and upper back with some shoulder rolls and head turns (see page 89). Drop your day from your shoulders and take a few relaxed breaths. Form a steeple shape with your hands by gently spreading your fingertips wide and touching the tip of each finger and thumb together at chest height in front of your body. Feel the pulse of your fingertips and the warmth there, noticing how this gesture brings a real presence to your mind. Next notice how the elevation of your fingertips is echoed by the structure of your mouth. Press the tip of your tongue to the roof of your mouth, feeling how the upper palate is like the steeple lifting skywards. There is a poise and peace here. Repeat the words: '*I am the architect of my life*' and breathe life and belief into this statement.

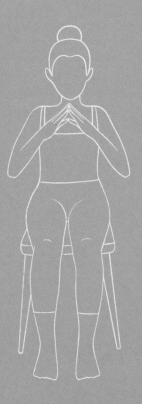

 Planting a seed: Each time you feel a longing for someone to rescue you, or the desire to avoid the current situation, remind yourself that you can stand tall. Ask yourself, where can you take action now? Even if the answers are not clear right now, they will come. Can you just sit with the uncertainty a while?

Recognize your foundations

As we embark on a new beginning often we feel we're at ground zero, or back to square one, and this can feel overwhelming. But remember, you're not building from scratch! Every life lesson learned, insight you've gleaned, strength you've developed and skill you've honed has laid the generous foundations and scaffolding for this next chapter of life, even if it is vastly different from the last. It is all transferable, relevant and applicable. You might like to jot down what some of these lessons are.

Meet your 'future best self'

As you feel a new identity forming, remember this a process rather than a destination. Your whole life long is one ceaseless process of becoming. Without putting any pressure on yourself, imagine your 'future best self'. As the current crush of life events resolves, who would you like to see rise from the ashes? What kind of choices do they make? How do they talk to themselves and others? How do they spend their time? You can do this in your mind's eye, journal about it, jot down words or phrases, doodle about it or cut out images and words and make a collage. See this incarnation of you come off the page, form a relationship with them in imagined conversations and draw on them for support and feedback.

 Planting a seed: In times of challenge, ask yourself, what would my 'future best self' do, tapping into your inner wisdom. Know that every decision you make in alignment with this vision takes you one step closer to being this version of you.

Decisions, decisions...

In forging a new path you may encounter a myriad of decisions. If you're facing a choice overload, see if you can reduce the number of options to get a clearer feel or reduce the number of choices you need to make right now. Do this in partnership with a friend if it feels overwhelming or go for a brisk walk and see if that brings greater clarity. Rather than feeling there is a 'right' or 'wrong' decision acknowledge that there can be several congruent options. It's not about making the one right choice, aim for a 'good' choice. How do you know what's a good choice? It will be harmonious with your values and it will draw on your strengths. You will also feel it in your body. When you're at peace with a choice, you'll sense it in your belly and your breath. If there is discord, your body will let you know, so listen to that gut feel. If you feel stuck in indecision it might help to set some timeframes and use these prompts:

- If I take this option, what are the benefits?

- If I don't take this path, what will I lose?

- How will I feel if I don't do this?

- What's motivating me – is it fear, doubt, the inner critic or is it hope, insight or courage?

- If a friend was facing this choice, what would I advise them?

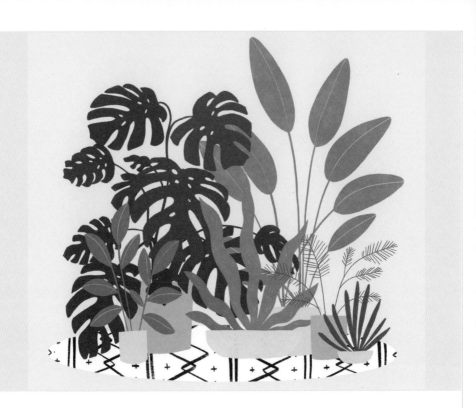

 Planting a seed: If you're feeling weighed down by a decision, tap into a sense of curiosity. It doesn't have to be an onerous task of finding the one right path. You don't have to have all the answers right away. Don't let doubt and the inner critic convince you it is too hard or that you don't know enough. Plant the seed, tenderly nurture it. Don't squash it with pressure and worries. Let it germinate and see what grows! There can be malleability too – try things out and if they don't take flight, we learn from the experience and grow. Try these mantras to support you in your decision making: *'I know myself'*, *'I am confident in myself'*, *'I trust my instincts'*, *'I have faith in my choices'*.

Draw on your team for support

Who on your team can help you in this new chapter? It can be powerful just saying out loud what you'd like to set in motion, forming a psychological contract to help keep you on track, a kind ear when you're tested and a warm hug to celebrate progress. Is there someone who's been through something similar who can walk the path with you? If there is something you'd like to do or achieve, can you reach out to someone doing that to find out about their journey? Maybe you'll need to look beyond your current circle and find someone or a group who can mentor you in this new stage of life, or if you feel moved, you could start your own support group or charitable venture to connect with kindred spirits. There is great zest and healing to be found in being of service to others.

Firing your arrow of intent – goals to help galvanize you

Once you have clarity on new directions, forming some goals will help you take action. The best kind of goals are deeply rooted in what you want for you, not what other people want for you. They are anchored in your values and you'll get clear on this when you consider 'why' you want to move in this direction. They are framed around what you want to do more of or become, rather than what you want to minimize or avoid. Your goals will need to complement not compete with each other. They will also need to take into consideration the variables at hand – time, energy and finances – and because these are constantly changing, your goals also need to be fluid to be realistic.

How to make sustainable habit change

- If there is some kind of change you'd like to make, first reflect on what you are currently doing. Bring your current choices to the light, examine their ramifications and ask yourself, what do you stand to lose if you keep doing the same things?

- Dig beneath what you want to change and ask yourself *why* you want to do things differently. It's your why that will serve you when temptation arises.

- For change to be sustainable we need to make it in small increments. Forget sweeping change that is hard to keep up, opt for waves of change. Address change by building one habit at a time. For example, with your eating, address one meal of the day at a time until it's on automatic pilot and then you're ready for the next wave of change.

Use your body to cultivate confidence and courage

Get out of your head and bring your plans to life using your body. While exploring these different shapes use ujjayi breathing (see page 165) to deepen your feeling of strength and resolve. You might also like to use the following mantras and observe how the postures give you a felt sense of these statements:

- *I have my own back.*

- *I am my own advocate.*

- *I honour my boundaries.*

- *I speak my truth.*

- *I am capable, resourceful, creative, strong, resilient or ready.*

- *I stand firm.*

- *Nothing will blow me off course.*

- *I know my 'why'.*

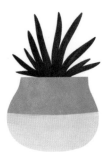

Mountain Side Bend, for energy and flexibility

Imagine you are standing between two panes of glass so you cannot arch or round your spine. All you can do is send roots down through your feet and reach up through your crown. Breathe in and raise your right arm, palm facing you. As you breath out, reach up and over to the left, banana shaping the right side of your body, and sliding your left hand down your left thigh. Breathe in and come back to upright, right arm skywards. Breathe out and allow your right arm to softly fall like a feather back down by your side. Repeat with the left arm and take three to six on each side, feeling your malleability and zest amplify.

Standing Dynamic Balance, for your core

Stand with your feet hip width apart, sense of humour engaged. As you breathe in raise your arms overhead and lift your right knee as high as you can, flexing your right heel. As you exhale, take your right arm back behind you, your left arm in front of you, both at shoulder height, and let your torso twist toward the right. If it's tricky to balance, keep looking forward, for extra challenge turn your gaze to the right. Breathe in and raise your arms overhead, looking forward. Exhale to bring your arms down and your right foot back to the floor. Repeat to the left and take three to six on each side, connecting with the strength of your stomach and the muscles that run along the length of your spine. This exercise is inherently difficult. Use it to develop awareness of 'right effort' – too little effort and we're floppy, too much effort and we become rigid. Find that sweet spot of right effort and it'll help you balance in this pose and in life in general.

Woodchopper Twist, for suppleness and release

Stand with your feet twice shoulder width apart, toes pointing forward, hands in prayer at your heart. Breathe in, stretch your hands up high and look up. Exhale, bend your right knee and bring your left elbow across your right thigh, keeping your neck long, hands firmly at your heart, torso twisting to the right. Breathe in, straighten your legs, raise your hands and look up, then twist to the left, using your elbow to lever your upper body deeper into the twist. Repeat three to six times each side, feeling how the twist allows you to see things from a different perspective. Notice how much taller you feel afterwards.

Dancer pose, for bravery

Standing tall, take your right ankle in your right hand. Keeping your hips and chest square, slowly explore taking your right leg back as if the foot is trying to escape your hand and reach your chest and your left hand forward. There's a real dynamic tension, moving both forward and backward, the front of your body elongating like a drawn bow. Feel the muscles of your back body engage and let this anchor you deep in the knowledge that you have your own back. Hold for five to ten smooth breaths, before repeating on the other side.

Wide Fold, Hang and Drape, to replenish

Stand with your feet twice shoulder width apart, toes pointing forward. Soften your knees and as you breathe out, hinge at your hips and take your fingertips toward the floor, bending your knees as much as necessary to allow this to be comfortable. Allow your spine to unfurl, head to hang, with the option of holding onto your elbows if this feels good. Stay for five breaths then drape yourself over your right leg, holding onto your right foot, ankle or knee, head toward your right toes for five to ten breaths. Repeat on the left then come back to the centre for another five breaths. Move straight to all fours or Child's pose (see page 136) to refresh, acknowledging there is a time for effort and a time for surrender.

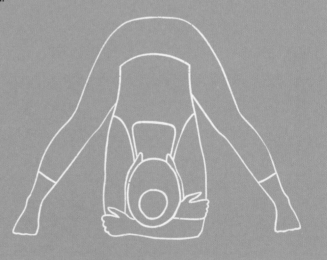

Downward Dog with hands out, feeling the strength and support of your back body

From all fours, raise your hips and press your heels back and down. Keep your knees soft if this allows you to better lengthen your spine. Feel how this works your arms and shoulder muscles. Now spin your fingertips to point outwards, noticing how this flattens your shoulder blades against your body, powerfully engaging your upper back muscles. Connect with this sensation of strength and support in the back of your body. For extra challenge, keep those muscles switched on as you slowly pivot your hands to point forward again. Five to ten breaths of work then sink into Child's pose (see page 136), softening, rounding and relaxing your upper back. Those muscles can soften and release but are strong and supportive when required. Remember that you can be your own safe place in softness and in strength.

Rest!

Your work is done. Lie on your front, back or take your legs up the wall, you choose. Let your comfort guide you. Enjoy five minutes of feeling your breath, softening your physical body or repeating a mantra that cultivates how you want to feel. Bask in the glow of this moment, feeling alive, feeling gratitude for this breath.

 Planting a seed: Notice how you can use your body, breath and mind to feel powerful and resourceful. In times of change and challenge, lift the crown of your head, slide your shoulder blades down, and feel the strength of your back. Know that you can advocate for yourself, taking action in service of your values.

When I feel lost or confused I'll...

- Hold my own hand or place my hands across my heart and repeat the words '*I am my own safe place*' or '*I feel my breath come home*'.

- Observe my thoughts, feelings and sensations, connecting with that part of me that witnesses these changing states.

- Remember it's ok to not have all the answers, or any of them! Clarity will come in time.

- Extend tenderness and kindness toward myself, turning to my Vitality Wheel for direction.

When I feel impatient or pressured I'll...

- Soften my body, relax my breath and repeat the words '*I have all the time I need*'.

- Check in with my goals, my diary for today and keep things small, focusing only on what I need to achieve today. Tomorrow can wait.

- Give myself a few minutes to reboot. There are diminishing returns for pushing through and a little relaxation can give me the peace and clarity I need.

When I feel stuck I'll...

- Consider whether forgiveness, acceptance or gratitude might free me.

- Draw on nature's beauty or a meditative shower to feel a shift of energy.

- Take the smallest action and see how this breaks inertia.

- Give myself the gift of time.

- Take some slow, relaxed mountain breaths (see page 134).

When I feel tempted I'll...

- Ask my 'future best self' what they would do.

- Call to mind my values and intentions, bearing in mind the consequences of giving in to this temptation. What do I stand to lose?

- Distract myself with something uplifting – scent, movement, nature, something funny.
- Call a buddy for support.
- Look at what lies beneath this impulse and address this deeper need with love and compassion.

When I know what I want but I don't know how I'll...

- Research how others have done similar things, listening to TED talks, podcasts or reading books.
- Talk to my support team and see what suggestions come up.
- Remember times I've felt this in the past and recognize that I can find my own solutions.
- Take comfort in knowing there isn't one right way, there can be several good options to try.
- Use the prompt: 'I wonder...'

When I want to feel courageous and strong I'll...

- Use my body to connect with my personal power, feeling the earth rise to support me, bringing my spine upright, shoulders down and gaze forward with intent.
- Repeat the words: '*I stand tall. I am capable. I have my own back*'.
- Take a few deep breaths or use ujjayi (see page 165) to galvanize me.
- Call to mind previous challenges I have overcome, connecting with my strengths, using them to navigate what lies ahead.
- Remember I don't have to be brave all the time, I can take time out to soothe when I need.

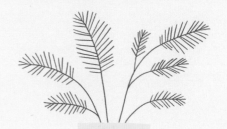

AFTERWORD

The silver lining to my struggle: I'll never again let a moment of peace pass me by unappreciated.

While the pages of this book are drawing to a close, our journey together continues. Please know I'm walking with you, side by side. Come back to this book, dipping in at will, the friend in your back pocket. This is a process and we're in it together. What leaped out at you on your first read will differ next time. There are layers to the skills and practices and with each read you'll integrate the insights deeper and find new ideas that pique your interest.

I hope you've found some solace here, that you feel a little calmer and less alone in the midst of what you're facing. I hope you feel more deeply and lovingly connected with your body, knowing that you can be your own safe place. I hope you feel more at peace with your emotions, allowing them to move through you, with tools to help you navigate the ones that can seem so hard to bear. I hope you feel more comfortable with change and transition, confident in your ability to evolve and to have your own back. I hope there is a resurgence of energy and faith that answers, clarity, a new sense of identity are all coming. *They are coming!* Just keep putting one foot in front of the other, knowing that you deserve to feel nourished and cared for. You matter. You are worthy of self-care and there really are no barriers to it. I hope you feel empowered with many nourishing things that you can do, unlocking that self-healing capacity you were born with.

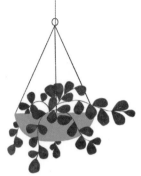

What next?

This is super simple, but we
often forget, we have to KEEP doing it. Even when you start
to feel lighter and brighter, don't let self-care slip away.
Hopefully it'll be embedded in the natural flow of your day
with your new skill set but keep paying in to your energy
bank with nourishing choices. The catch cry of those
relapsing into energetic bankruptcy is 'oh, I forgot about
it...I used to do that...I was feeling great so didn't think I
needed it any more'. Life keeps happening, so self-care
needs to keep happening.

And when you do forget it or drop it and you wind up flat
on your back again, just learn from it. We've all been there
too. Dust yourself off with tenderness. You know what to
do. One micro-moment of self-care at a time. Maybe next
time you'll catch yourself before you fall. Notice how much
faster you got back on your feet this time.

As we've been journeying through this book together,
look at how far you've come. Please celebrate that
development. Maybe you've not quite reached where you
want to be just yet, but there is time! There will still be
accomplishments to reflect on, effort to commend, and
that celebration might just give you the zest to take that
next step. Mine those silver linings and carry on! We learn
and grow together and I am willing you on.

REFERENCES

[1] Sarah Marsh and Amanda Boateng, 'Quarter of 14-year-old girls in UK have self-harmed, report finds', the *Guardian*, 29 August 2019.

[2] digital.nhs.uk, 'Mental Health of Children and Young People in England, 2017', 22 November 2018.

[3] Ons.gov.uk, 'Suicides in the UK: 2018 registrations'.

[4] Tommys.org, 'Suicide is the leading cause of death in new mothers', 1 November 2018.

[5] Jayashri Kulkarni, 'Perimenopausal depression – an under-recognised entity', *Australian Prescriber* 41 (6): 183–185, 3 December 2018.

[6] Bessel van der Kolk, *The Body Keeps the Score* (London: Penguin 2014).

[7] Peter A Levine, *In an Unspoken Voice: How the Body Releases Trauma and Restores Goodness* (New York: North Atlantic Books 2010).

[8] Ibid.

[9] Stephen Porges Lecture 'Polyvagal Theory, Oxytocin and the Neurobiology of Love and Trust', 8 June 2019, London.

[10] Bessel Ven Der Kolk, *The Body Keeps the Score* (London: Penguin 2014).

[11] Mentalhealth.org.uk, 'Let's Get Physical', 2013.

[12] Erik Peper, I-Mei Lin, Richard Harvey, Jacob Perez, 'How Posture Affects Memory Recall and Mood', *Biofeedback* vol. 45, issue 2, pp. 36–41.

[13] Erik Peper, '"Don't slouch!" Improve health with posture feedback', peperperspective.com, 1 July 2019.

[14] Erik Peper, I-Mei Lin, 'Increase or Decrease Depression: How Body Postures Influence Your Energy Level', *Biofeedback* vol. 40, issue 3, pp. 125–30.

[15] Dr Libby Weaver, 'Rushing woman's syndrome', YouTube.com, 29 August 2012.

[16] Arjun Walia, 'Big Pharma CEO: "My Primary Responsibility is to Shareholders"', Collective-evolution.com, 1 October 2019.

[17] Juliete Tocino-Smith, 'What is Eustress and How is it Different than Stress?', Positivepsychology.com, 25 October 2019.

[18] Christian Jarrett, 'What's your stress mindset?', *British Psychological Society Research Digest*, 5 January 2018.

[19] Daeun Park et al, 'Beliefs About Stress Attenuate the Relation Among Adverse Life Events, Perceived Distress, and Self-Control', Child Development, vol. 89, issue 6, November/December 2018.

[20] Juliete Tocino-Smith, 'What is Eustress and How is it Different than Stress?', Positivepsychology.com, 25 October 2019.

[21] Kelly McGonigal, 'How to make stress your friend', TEDGlobal 2013, ted.com.

[22] Elizabeth D Kirby, Sandra E Muroy, Wayne G Sun, David Covarrubias, Megan J Leong, Laurel A Barchas and Daniela Kaufer, 'Acute stress enhances adult rat hippocampal neurogenesis and activation of newborn neurons via secreted astrocytic FGF2', *eLife* 2013; 2: e00362.

[23] Bruce Goldman, 'Study explains how stress can boost immune system', med.stanford.edu, 21 June 2012.

[24] K Asbacher, A O'Donovan, O M Wolkowitz, F S Dhabhar, Y Su, E Epel, 'Good stress, bad stress and oxidative stress: insights from anticipatory cortisol reactivity', *Psychoneuroendocrinology*, September 2013; 38(9): 1698–708.

[25] Ibid.

[26] Shawn Achor, 'The Right Kind of Stress Can Bond Your Team Together', *Harvard Business Review*, 14 December 2015.

[27] Herbert J Freudenberger and Geraldine Richelson, *Burnout: The High Cost of High Achievement* (New York: Anchor 1980).

[28] Christina Maslach et al, Maslach Burnout Inventory, mindgarden.com.

[29] Britta K. Holzel et al, 'Mindfulness practice leads to increases in regional brain gray matter density', *Psychiatry Research: Neuroimaging*, vol. 191, issue 1, 30 January 2011.

[30] Timothy D Wilson et al, 'Just think: The challenges of the disengaged mind', *Science*, 4 July 2014, vol. 345, issue 6192.

[31] **Erik Peper**, 'Toning quiets the mind and increases HRV more quickly than mindfulness practice', peperperspective.com, adapted from Peper et al, 'Which quiets the mind more quickly and increases HRV: Toning or mindfulness?', *Neuroregulation* 6(3) 2019.

[32] **Adrian F Ward et al**, 'Brain Drain: The Mere Presence of One's Own Smartphone Reduces Available Cognitive Capacity', *Journal for the Association of Consumer Research*, vol. 2, no. 2, April 2017.

[33] **Trevor Haynes**, 'Dopamine, Smartphones and You: A battle for your time', Harvard University blog, 1 May 2018.

[34] **Leslie J Seltzer et al**, 'Social vocalization can release oxytocin in humans', Proceedings of the Royal Society of Biological Sciences, 12 May 2010.

[35] **Kyle J Bourassa et al**, 'The impact of physical proximity and attachment working models on cardiovascular reactivity: Comparing mental activation and romantic partner presence', *Psychopsychology*, 4 January 2019.

[36] **Erika Jackson**, 'Stress Relief: The role of exercise in stress management', *ACSM's Health and Fitness Journal*, May/June 2013, vol. 17 issue 3.

[37] **Carol Dweck**, 'The power of believing you can improve', TEDxNorrkoping, November 2014, ted.com.

[38] **Patrice Voss et al**, 'Dynamic Brains and the Changing Rules of Neuroplasticity: Implications for Learning and Recovery', *Frontiers in Psychology*, 2017; 8: 1657.

[39] **Elisabeth Kübler-Ross and David Kessler**, *On Grief and Grieving: Finding the Meaning of Grief Through the Five Stages of Loss* (London: Simon & Schuster 2014).

[40] **Jenny Florence**, 'What is Emotional Health?', huffpost.com. https://www.huffpost.com/entry/what-is-emotional-health_b_6023648

[41] **Susan David**, *Emotional Agility: Get Unstuck, Embrace Change, and Thrive in Work and Life* (New York: Penguin Random House 2016).

[42] **Lisa Feldman Barrett**, 'Emotional Intelligence Needs a Rewrite', *Nautilus*, 3 August 2017.

[43] **Lisa Feldman Barrett et al**, 'Knowing what you're feeling and knowing what to do about it: Mapping the relation between emotion differentiation and emotion regulation', *Cognition and Emotion*, vol. 15 2001, issue 6.

[44] **Todd B Kashdan et al**, 'Emotion Differentiation as Resilience Against Excessive Alcohol Use: An Ecological Momentary Assessment in Underage Social Drinkers', *Psychological Science*, 9 August 2010.

[45] **Richard S Pond Jr et al**, 'Emotion differentiation moderates aggressive tendencies in angry people: A daily diary analysis', *Emotion*, vol. 12 (2), April 2012.

[46] https://www.brainyquote.com/citation/quotes/helen_keller_133193

[47] **Alexandra Sacks**, 'A new way to think about the transition to motherhood', TED Residency 2018, ted.com.

[48] **Emma Young**, 'Our Golden Years? Research Into The Ups And Downs Of Retirement, Digested', *British Psychological Society Digest*, 9 October 2019.

[49] **William Bridges**, *Transitions: Making Sense of Life's Changes* (New York: Da Capo Press 2004).

[50] **D L MacInnes**, 'Self-esteem and self-acceptance: an examination into their relationship and their effect on psychological health.', *Journal of Psychiatric and Mental Health Nursing*, October 2006; 13(5):483–9.

[51] **Anant Narayan Sinha et al**, 'Assessment of the Effects of Pranayama/Alternate Nostril Breathing on the Parasympathetic Nervous System in Young Adults', *Journal of Clinical and Diagnostic Research*, May 2013; 7(5): 821–823.

[52] **Jitendra Mahour and Pratibha Verma**, 'Effect of Ujjayi Pranayama on cardiovascular autonomic function tests', *National Journal of Physiology, Pharmacy and Pharmacology*, 9 December 2016.

[53] **Richard G. Tedeschi, Jane Shakespeare-Finch, Kanako Taku and Lawrence G Calhoun**, *Posttraumatic Growth* (London: Routledge 2018).

INDEX

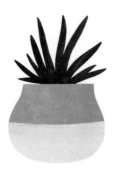

Index

ACKNOWLEDGEMENTS

Deepest thanks to my darling husband Dave, for being there for me every step of the way, lifting me up in difficult times, always championing me and celebrating the fruits of our labour together. To Charlotte and Ted, thank you for being the light in every day, filling me up. I'm grateful to my mum for walking with me even when we're oceans apart. Thank you to my buddies Donna, Nikki, Charlotte, Danielle, Clare and Emma for your medicinal humour and care. This book is very much a collective achievement and I am so grateful to Jane Graham Maw, Becky Anderson and the team at Aster for not only making this book possible but for working so hard to make it available when it's most needed – heartfelt thanks to Kate Adams, Pauline Bache, Yasia Williams, Megan Brown, Hazel O'Brien, Melissa Baker and Alice Groser. I am also grateful to Madeline Kate Martinez for bringing this book to life with her deeply nourishing art.